Gut Feelings

A guide for Crohn's and Colitis patients

Rafael Moreno

Gut Feelings

A guide for Crohn's and Colitis patients

Fourth edition – 2015

Produced in co-operation with The Israeli Association for the Support of Crohn's Disease and Intestinal Colitis Patients

Medical advice:

Dr Nitzan Maharshak, Inflammatory Bowel Disease Unit, Gastro Institute, Ichilov Hospital

Translation to English:

Paul Clingman

Language editing:

Yif'al Bistari

Einat Kedem

Cover design:

Hili Chiko

Editing:

Rafael Moreno

Message from the Association

One would assume that every Crohn's disease or Colitis patient would be aware of the benefits stemming from the ever-widening knowledge of the disease – its causes, its course, and the possibilities available for treatment – possibilities that are developing and increasing without pause. However this awareness is not an easy thing for many of us. There are those who are not interested in knowing and prefer to ignore matters. A mechanism of repression such as this may help them to distance themselves from dealing with the disease, but in the long term it can bring disastrous results that are hard to put right.

There are others who find themselves swamped with information on the internet. This information does not dispel the concerns and fears – not least because of the difficulty of deciding whether the sources are reliable. In many cases these doubts lead to even more intensive surfing and real fears.

One of the important challenges facing The Israeli Association for the Support of Crohn's Disease and Intestinal Colitis Patients lies in overcoming these difficulties – not just for those who have chosen to repress their fears, and for those surfers who have not managed to find answers to their concerns, but also for those to whose hearts we have not yet found a way. In his book, Rafael Moreno, who is a member of the Association, presents a correct balance in the various approaches to the disease, and because of that, he is the bearer of truly good news. The book describes Rafael's personal means of coping with the disease, and in doing so, it equips the reader with knowledge and useful and important wisdom from the perspective of someone who has experienced the disease himself. The book supplies important tools for dealing with the disease on a daily basis, and carries a message of optimism and a better future.

The Israeli Association for the Support of Crohn's Disease and Intestinal Colitis Patients is proud to have the opportunity of participating in the production of this book and sees in it an important means of support for patients and their families.

Disclaimer

The information that appears in this book is of a general nature only. It makes no claim to present professional opinions or certified professional or medical advice. You may not use the information that appears in this book for the purpose of self-diagnosis or treatment. It is incumbent upon the reader to seek an opinion or medical advice before making any use of the information that appears in this book. The information in this book is not a substitute for the professional advice of a doctor. Acting upon the advice in this book is the responsibility of the reader alone. The author of this book bears no responsibility of any kind, for any damage (direct or indirect) that might be caused, or deemed to be caused arising as a result of the use of the information presented in this book. The author is not responsible for any errors, inaccuracies or omissions in the book. Any errors that might occur are inadvertent.

I would love to hear your comments:
iGutFeelings@gmail.com

Gut Feelings on the Web:
igutfeelings.com

Dedicated to my family that helps me in difficult times.

Contents

Introduction

In 1995 I was diagnosed with Crohn's disease. The doctors explained that the stomach pains that I had recently been experiencing as well as the tiredness, temperatures and diarrhea, were all symptoms of the disease. They added that it was a chronic inflammatory disease of the digestive system that mainly affects the intestines.

"What do I do?" I asked.
"Don't eat fresh fruit and vegetables or spicy foods, and take pills every day," they replied.
"And what else?"
"That's it, more or less… Good luck."

The first thing that crossed my mind was that it was true that for a long time I had diarrhea and had been tired. It seemed that I had learned to live with it. Okay – so at least now I have a certificate and I'm not a hypochondriac. There was almost no information about the disease itself. I therefore assumed that nothing would happen if I were to continue living and eating normally. When I used to eat junk food, I would go a little more often to the toilet. So what? I was used to it.

It was only five years later in the city of Cuzco in Peru when I had my first real attack, that I began to understand in the most trying way that this matter that needed a little more attention.

Today I'm thirty-five years old. In the twenty years since I was diagnosed as a Crohn's patient, I tried nearly every possible medication for the disease. I was treated by tens of alternative practitioners with various approaches, and went through countless check-ups and one operation. And it was after the operation that I decided to write this book in order to help Crohn's patients avoid reaching the point at which surgical intervention is required.

During the years I have gathered experience that today helps me take more enlightened decisions with regard to my lifestyle and the ways of handling my disease. At the end of the day, every patient needs to consider independently for himself questions such as which medications to consume, what to eat, where to work, or whether to undergo an operation. If I could have had the benefit of others' knowledge and experience twenty years ago, there is no doubt that I would not have needed the operation. If I had been aware of the extraordinary difficulties that my body would find itself in as a result of the disease – a disease that at the outset doesn't seem particularly threatening – I would have done anything to avoid them.

Crohn's disease does not bode the end of the world. It's definitely possible to live with it. The question is what the quality of that life will be – in other words, to what degree can the patient live a normal life?

I have never thought of not living my life the way I want to, despite those periods when I suffered badly from the disease. Over the years I've learned to understand the limitations imposed by the disease and to live within their bounds. The wiser I became in living my life more correctly, the less apparent the disease became. My quality of life improved and the framework of my capabilities widened. During my years as a Crohn's patient I have managed to travel, to finish my studies in electrical engineering at Tel Aviv University, to marry, and even to turn into a young father. Today I work full-time at a company that works in program development. Of course this doesn't necessarily mean that my condition only ever improves. My life is a series of ups and downs. But I learn from my own experience all the time, and do my best to monitor the status of my health on a continuous basis.

My personal experience and the research I've done demonstrate two main points concerning the information that is given to the Crohn's patient about the disease. The first is the lack of certified information. It's true that the internet has created a revolution that led to the instantaneous sharing of knowledge on an immense scale. In fact, today every patient can be helped in forums and other sites to search for information on his disease and various means of treatment. Having said that, stories and advice from patients in internet chats cannot cover for the lack of certified information, whether it be on the internet or at a clinic close to your home. As close as personal stories may be to that of an anonymous patient thirsty for any piece of information and advice, they cannot diagnose his disease, and cannot recommend its correct treatment. This is especially true when dealing with incurable diseases, like Crohn's disease, that force the patients to pursue alternative treatments and compel them to adjust to an unfamiliar lifestyle.

If the one side of the problem is the lack of certified information, then the other is an abundance of false information. This kind of information is partially caused by people who in all innocence want to help, but do not know how. They might be relatives, or merely acquaintances who experienced abdominal upsets at the end of the sixties, something that has conferred on them honorary doctorates in various gastroenterological diseases. Alternatively they might be practitioners who have completed a two-week advanced study course that has given them the ability to heal you of any disease. The second aspect of the false information arises from various greedy people like those who will sell you potions, treatments and any other thing they feel like to achieve one thing – money. False information can reach you in every possible way – especially if you are desperate for answers and are experiencing the darkness of the lack of knowledge. Where the false information comes from makes absolutely no difference.

What is important is to identify it. If, God forbid, you allow it to confuse you, the monetary damage will be child's play compared with the damage to your health.

The aim of this book is to bring you the information that I have gathered from my own experience and from in-depth research that includes interviews with many highly-esteemed professionals. It is meant to give tools to the patient to deal with the disease, and with the decisions that need to be taken throughout life as a result of it. I have done my best to use simple language as far as possible so that even the younger among us will be able to follow and understand. The humor that runs though many parts of the book is not there just to provide enjoyment in the reading. It is actually an inseparable part of the positive approach that patients need to adopt in order to improve the state of their health. Naturally no-one should infer from it any disregard or recklessness concerning the seriousness of the disease. I know as well as anyone how much suffering can be caused by it. At the same time it provides many situations which, if you were not personally involved in them, would seem extremely funny.

The book deals mainly with Crohn's disease. After all, that is the disease that I know (and love). At the same time, I'm certain that most of the information that appears in it can serve patients of other intestinal diseases like Colitis that is also an incurable chronic inflammatory disease with symptoms and methods of treatment that greatly resemble those of Crohn's disease.

This book is intended for you as a Crohn's or Colitis patient, and for your family members who help you to deal with it. The information in it is not intended to be a substitute for the professional advice of a treating doctor, but rather to be a gateway to existing information about the disease. It has been written in the hope that it will be useful in helping you to make better choices concerning your nutrition, lifestyle, therapist and alternative medical treatment that suits you and to provide you with sources of information upon which you can rely. Apart from this you will be able to learn about the approach of western conventional medicine to Crohn's disease and Colitis and their diagnosis and methods of treatment.

I am certain that by the time they have finished reading it, every family member will know more about the character of the disease that the patient has to deal with, and that every patient will have a growing sense that it is within his or her power to improve their health.

Every word of what follows has been written in blood, sweat and not a little gas.

Enjoy.

My first time

My first real encounter with Crohn's disease was in Peru, in a town called Cuzco.

I was twenty years old and wanting to see the world. Perhaps it would be more correct to say that what I really wanted was to go out and have fun. It didn't really matter to me in which country, or which language was being spoken around me. The main thing was that it should all be cheap and cool. It was after a two-month tour of Ecuador and Peru that we arrived in Cuzco. As a great devotee of sea and sun, I was by that stage pretty fed up with the mountains, the cold and the general air of inaction that prevailed up there.

But what could you do when, as the locals and the tourists unanimously claimed, you absolutely "had to see" Machu Picchu, that ancient Peruvian city built on a mountain.
Well, if you absolutely had to see it, well then, you had to see it.

So instead of travelling for half a day and escaping to Brazil as so many good people tend to do, we decided – our group of five Israelis – to spend the night in the field, as part of a two-day tour up the mountain.

The people responsible for organizing the expedition were from a Peruvian tour company, a fact which by this stage of my trip, should definitely have rung alarm bells. I had already had all kinds of dubious experiences with Peruvians during the previous month, in which the exactitude of any agreement was at the very least certain not to extend to details.

Our agreement with the company for this trip was that they would supply an English-speaking guide, food for the full two days, and a means of transport for the journey back, which was to include a bus trip down the mountain, a train journey, and yet another four-hour leg back to the city. And as for us? Well, all we were expected to do was come along and enjoy the view.

After checking a number of companies, undertaking some brief research among experienced tourists and doing some quick bargaining about prices, we set off. Already at our first get-together with the guide it was very clear that his English vocabulary did not comprise much more than the word "hello." Also, the sight of his tiny bag which was meant to contain enough food to stave off the hunger of six people for the entire tour, did nothing to add to any sense of calm.

The trip began with a climb that was not especially difficult, and its route took in some very interesting sites. If only we'd remembered to bring along a translator or a English-Spanish dictionary, we might have understood why.

Because our amigo was carrying all the provisions by himself, and was making such an effort to explain the heritage of his land to us, at a certain point we stopped cutting him short in the midst of the explanations he was giving at every stop. We simply let him continue explaining various subjects that appeared – at least to him – to be very important. In this way he managed to stretch the excursion out over the entire day.

I, who have never been thought of as a big eater, feel the sensation of hunger relatively quickly (possibly because I don't have any great reserves). Very soon thoughts of food were the only things that were going through my mind and my stomach.

I should point out that in the light of my bitter experience with Peruvians I did display a little responsibility, in that I had bought a few crackers and nuts just in case the culinary aspect of this trip would turn out to be somewhat less satisfactory than expected. Responsible or not – by midday, after a half a day of trekking, I found myself with an empty backpack and an even emptier stomach.

I came to the conclusion that if I wanted to reach the camp where we were due to spend the night – and even more importantly, to receive our evening meal – then I needed to calm myself down and not waste any more energy on our talented guide.

Our sublime lunch turned out to be a wing-and-a-half of chicken for each hiker – a morsel which on a normal day I wouldn't even think of giving to my dog. But on that particular day – which was far from being normal – I was literally licking my fingers.

After another few hours that seemed to take an eternity, the evening meal finally materialized. By then I wasn't interested in what was on the plate. Despite the threatening growls of my table companions about the somewhat suspicious look of the steak, I completely cleaned my plate. I did however refrain from asking for more.

I was a bit disappointed with myself because during the first two months of the trip I had been careful not eat any kind of meat out of fear of an undesirable response on the part of my stomach. It's known, however, that it's not just an army that marches on its stomach. Another full day of hiking awaited me on the ascent up the mountain, without any comprehensible guidance or explanation or break for lunch.

And there was evening and there was morning – the second day of hiking.

I woke in the morning with unfamiliar feelings in my stomach. If I hadn't become knowledgeable about Crohn's disease over the previous five years and the way it manifests with diarrhea, anemia and other symptoms, I would have said that it felt like a real pain.

I didn't get too excited, and I walked to the place where up to that point I had solved all similar problems – the bathroom. And the more I sat and thought, and sat again, and thought again, I understood that there was nothing left of the steak of the night before – and that there was no movement down south. And at the same time, the pain was just getting worse. It was at that point that I understood that I had a problem: Here I was in the middle of nowhere with completely new sensations, and with a journey of at least a day ahead of me, before I could hope to reach any sign of civilization (Peruvian, perhaps, but still – civilization).

I couldn't really depend on the guide for anything, and waiting for some rescue didn't seem to me to be a prudent idea – and in any case it would probably arrive in the form of an exhausted donkey.

I decided to try my luck at the summit of the mountain – after all how bad could it be?

The rest of the day was supposed to include a guided tour of a few hours in Machu Picchu , and after that would come the three-part journey back to Cuzco. In the early hours, after I had assessed the state of my health, I decided that the challenge was not too great, and that I should continue the journey. At the same time I didn't feel it was necessary to update my friends. Uncalled-for pressure wouldn't help anybody. It was enough that one tourist was stressed.

At that time, all I knew about Crohn's disease was what I had experienced before – diarrhea and tiredness. That was enough for me – perhaps because I believed that there are things that it's better not to know. What I did know was that the disease could cause adhesions of the bowel, something that would be characterized by a hard and swollen stomach, symptoms that I had already identified that day. Although I was really worried, I continued on the journey back – without any clue of what I would do when I eventually returned to the city.

The pain and the swelling, as well as the general sensation that the food was stuck, brought me to the conclusion that eating now would not be the best idea. I decided to drink a lot in the hope that that would get me through the day. During the journey to the lost city I felt all right, even though the pain was constantly growing. When we reached the ruins I rested on a rock while the guide delivered a long and learned explication of the place.

In the afternoon when we reached the large parking area for buses where the tourists had gathered I tried my luck again in the bathroom, but didn't make any progress. At this point I started to feel under pressure, something that only made the pains in my stomach worse. The truth is I simply didn't know what to do.

I convinced myself to calm down and continue – not that I had any choice. We boarded the bus after a period of preparation that seemed to last an eternity, and we descended the mountain on the road to the train station. At the foot of the mountain it turned out that the train would only arrive in a few hours, and considering the dump that we found ourselves in I felt that despite the feeling that I was going to explode at any moment the right thing to do would be to try and nap on the grass. The hours passed but the pain remained and even worsened, and as could be expected, the train was packed and the journey felt endless. The truth is, that in my state, every move took an eternity.

We arrived at the train station in the evening. The nearest city was at least a four-hour journey away. I was suffering from intolerable pain, and I had not eaten since six that morning. I sat down on a bench at the station, while all around me was the chaos, crush and noise of tired tourists and locals with goods and giant loads on their backs. As I sat I felt that this was it. I was not going to move from here. At this point, as I was sinking into self-pity. I tried not to panic when I was informed that no-one was waiting for us at the station, and that we would have to find another way to get back.

After another eternity or two that probably only took an hour, it was decided that we would get into some kind of communal taxi that could accommodate our whole group as well as an amount of locals who could have populated a medium-sized country. On the way my situation just got worse. At about ten at night, when there were still two hours to go on the journey, I felt that I could not carry on and I asked the driver to pull over. There, in the middle of nowhere, on the grass at the side of the road, and with the taxi full of tourists and Peruvians behind me, for the second time I made the acquaintance of something I hadn't seen for a full day – the steak and its extras. For some very long moments I could not stop throwing up my entire soul. I thought I was dying, but to my sorrow, the gods of Crohn were not going to give up on me so quickly. After I stopped throwing up, I drank a little water, washed my face, and calmed down. I returned to the taxi and did my best to hold on till the end of the journey.

After two hours the driver stopped in the center of the city. I sat down on the sidewalk and said to my friends that I was not moving from there, and that they should call an ambulance. I remember the surprise on their faces. After all – I had not said anything all day, and had given no hint of my situation. Since no-one had any idea how or even where to call an ambulance I was convinced to get into a taxi to go back to the hotel. When we got there, I didn't even go up to the room. I vomited my soul up in the toilets in the lobby, and although I thought that I had already seen all the items on the menu of the glorious meal of steak, the vomit reflex proved me wrong.

The hotel owner called an ambulance which arrived a few minutes later, and it took me, accompanied by two friends, to the hospital, a kind of private clinic mainly for tourists.

Because I didn't know exactly what I was suffering from, and because I didn't know the names of the drugs that could relieve the problem, I was at the mercy of the Peruvian doctor.

The first stage of the program was to give me painkillers, something for which I could only be thankful. After that two doctors examined me: The first, a likeable gastroenterologist, explained to me that it was simply the progression of the disease, and that it was essential that we treat this current attack. (This was to be the last time I would see this doctor for reasons which would become clear afterwards.) In contrast to him, however, there was the second doctor, who claimed that because the pain was on the right side of the lower abdomen, it meant that I was in fact suffering from appendicitis. Because of the danger, according to him, of the appendix bursting, it was necessary to do an urgent operation. He even added that in a case like this it was dangerous to wait, and that there was no possibility of flying to another city because there was a real fear that the situation would worsen. (Just in case I was thinking of fleeing that night, God forbid.)

His words aroused my suspicions, especially since I was beginning to get used to the addictive relief of the painkillers. There wasn't a lot of time to think. I was taken by one of the male nurses for an X-ray that required me to stand up – an exercise that didn't exactly combine perfectly with the painkillers I had received not long before. The next thing I remembered was a guy I didn't know trying to stabilize me, and then myself waking up in a bed. A period of time that seemed to me just seconds, had in fact lasted for about two hours of unconsciousness. It turned out that during this time the doctor from the first clinic had tried to get one of the girls I was touring with to sign an authorization for an operation to remove my appendix. Luckily for me she was in no hurry to sign. She had even called her mother who had once undergone a similar operation, and she had warned her not to sign anything.

When I woke up I didn't have the faintest clue about the owner's desire to operate on me so that he could earn as much money as possible from the insurance company. In retrospect it turned out that with my abdomen in an acute state, the operation could have seriously endangered me. During the night the "appendicitis doctor" came back to examine me. Fat and threatening, a man fleshy from feeding on a good few ripe appendixes for breakfast, and laden with rings and gold chains, the "doctor" pressured me to decide quickly: "We have to operate now. Time is running out."

Although the pain had lessened a little, it was still strong, and my stomach was hard and swollen. What was I to do? The appendicitis doctor left me no choice. All that was left was the last thing that any tourist wants to do: To call his parents and to worry them to death.

In my case it was definitely time for a second opinion from my specialist attending doctor – dad.

I made the call home, and I was praying, out of a desire to prevent panic, that my dad would answer. Mom picked up.

I said "Mom...! How are things...? Is everything all right? Me...? Okay... well, the truth is... my stomach's a little sore, I'm in hospital. There's a doctor here who wants to take out my appendix. Here, speak to him." I handed the phone to the doctor. My mother's response was "Okay, so come home." The minute the initial shock at home passed, I spoke to my father, and to the displeasure of the doctor it was decided that I would get through the night with antibiotics.

Two months later, in Israel, in discussions around the dinner table, it was explained to me that these had been critical hours. If it had been appendicitis, my condition would have deteriorated. If it had improved a little, then it would have been a flare-up of Crohn's disease. As you can imagine, the pressure they felt at home during those hours had been enormous. By the morning my situation had improved. There were less stomach pains, and less swelling and hardness.

I reported this to the family in Israel, and the situation calmed down a little. It wasn't like that with the appendicitis doctor and the owner of the clinic who continued with their "must operate urgently." This time, though, they backed up their diagnosis with an ultrasound test.

Days went by, with the pain lessening from day to day. After a week during which I barely ate a thing, it was decided that my condition was good enough for me to be discharged with all the internal organs with which I had been admitted.

With some trepidation I boarded a plane bound for the main airport in Peru's capital Lima , and from there I continued to the Israeli embassy. The flight passed without incident, and I met the embassy doctor at the central hospital. In an additional ultrasound test, it still wasn't clear whether it was an inflammation of the appendix, or another complication of Crohn's disease. At this point I decided to return to Israel, despite my original plan that had included another two months of touring.

After a conversation with my parents, in which they convinced me to continue touring (and for this I thank them from the bottom of my heart), I decided to give up on the mountains and the cold of Bolivia in favor of the sea and the heat of Brazil. I continued on a tour of surfing that included only good food and sporting activities, without the generous help of any drugs. My condition continued to improve wonderfully. By the time I had been back in Israel for two months, I had already put on about seven kilos more than my weight when I had left for my trip. With a disease like mine, we were talking about a kind of miracle, especially given the state that I had reached.

My first time was perfect proof of the real capacity of Crohn's disease. I understood for the first time just how much my condition could deteriorate if I didn't take care of my health. Perhaps even more importantly I learned that my body had the ability to heal itself, or at the very least, to bring about a marked improvement. Brazil, with the calm and relaxing atmosphere that it offered, the excellent food and sporting activities on the amazing beaches, had been the perfect setting for strengthening the body and calming the soul.

The operation

The preparatory period

In my twenties I had visitations of pains that included acute stomach pains, a "hard stomach" shivers, vomiting and fever. During this period my main concerns were finishing my electrical engineering degree, moving to my own apartment, and occupying an interesting full-time position at an interesting high-tech company.

Because the pains showed no sign of disappearing I accepted the recommendation of my attending doctor to begin a course of drugs that included steroids. Since the first attack, and up to that point, I had avoided drugs like that despite the recommendations of the doctors. However, soon enough I began to understand that I didn't really have a choice. If I was still interested in reaching all the goals that I had set for myself, I would need help. And with the help seeming so friendly and unthreatening (what could be threatening in tiny pink pills...?) the world appeared absolutely wonderful! I began taking the pills at the beginning of my fourth and last year of studies.

Almost immediately it became clear to me that all the wonderful stories that I had been told about steroids were true. I felt excellent. I went back to eating larger portions of food. I was full of energy, and felt able to do whatever I wanted in life just like every normal person. To my great disappointment this recipe for a normal life was limited to two months. And after that, in accordance with the doctor's instructions, I had to stop. Thus, after two magic months, exactly as my packed semester reached its climax, and in tandem with the hard work that was supposed to finance the rent, I tried (I really tried!) to stop or at least to lessen the dose of the steroids. My old friend from long ago was waiting for exactly this moment, Crohn's disease, which stormed back into my life at full tilt. Not only could I not stop popping the wonder drug, but there were even days when I could not help taking an extra (little) pill.

The days passed in this way, and once every two weeks I would try to reduce the dose, but without success. After a year, I found myself taking the same amount of steroids, but with attacks that came back, despite the pills. Inspired by the well-known saying – what doesn't work with force will work with more force – the doctor suggested a magical solution: Dear Rafael, I will increase the dose and move to a stronger type of steroid.

It can be said to my credit that at this point I did stop, and for the first time in a long time I really began to think about my situation. If I were to continue along the path of the wonder pills, where would it lead? What would happen in another year? And what, in two years…? With what daily dose of steroids would I have to equip my body in order to go to work, or just to get through the day without pain? And thus, from the one familiar (more or less) problem of Crohn's disease, another problem was added: I was addicted to steroids!

For the reader who is not familiar with the secret of the world of steroids, this may be the time for a short explanation about them and the way they work. Before anything else, it's important to note that despite all the advances in medicine it's still not known in any clear or exact way just how steroids affect the body. Among the few things that are known for certain is the fact that continued regular consumption is likely to endanger health, and to cause even more serious problems than the ones that the steroids are meant to solve. (I'll expand on this subject later on.)

According to what was explained to me by a wise doctor, the steroids create a kind of masking. Besides the quick physical improvement, they are also likely to prevent the patient from feeling the pain whose purpose is to warn of an impaired state of health. And it's true that I remembered that after one of the strongest attacks that I had experienced I was injected with a generous portion of steroids. From a prone position, desperate and suffering from unspeakable pain, I went almost immediately to running around on the beach, surfing and big meals, and in the following twenty-four hours I felt I was at peak fitness. (It strongly reminded me of the beginning of the film Requiem for a Dream.)

My unqualified advice, patient-to-patient, is to avoid as far as possible the taking of any steroids. While you can use them during difficult periods, avoid reaching a point of dependency. From the outset it is desirable to limit your use to a specified period. If God forbid you do get to the point of dependency, you simply have to rehabilitate yourself with determination. Apart from the fact that you will have to increase the dosage of the drugs – something that will increase your dependency on them and take you even further from a real solution for the disease – the problem will only get worse. The steroids will mask the signs of the disease and will convince you that it has disappeared. As a result of this you are likely to ignore your body's special needs, and pay no attention to the necessity of adapting to the eating habits and lifestyle required by a person in your condition. And when you succeed in the end in "beating the drug" you will discover that your condition has not improved, and often has even worsened as a result of your flawed lifestyle and nutrition.

But back to the story. When I understood that my condition was getting worse in tandem with my taking huge amounts of steroids, I decided to leave my work and my apartment to lessen the stresses in my life. I was hoping to rehabilitate myself from the steroids and to improve the state of my health. During my last period of exams, which included seven exams and a project, I could say that I was "clean". The condition of my body, however, was as bad as anything I had ever experienced. With my last strength, amidst frequent attacks, this nightmarish period also came to an end, an ending that left me mentally and physically drained. I understood that it was in reality impossible to continue. It seemed that it was only then that I truly began to internalize the fact that I had this disease called Crohn's – and to understand that this issue is a problem that you simply cannot ignore. I thought that the solution would come with time. And this time arrived very quickly, when after completing all my academic obligations I planned to start working. It was clear to me that before I could commit to a new place of work, I would have to improve the state of my health.

It was with a lot of motivation that I began to implement the plan: A complete break from all the drugs; an attempt to concentrate on healing the disease with the help of alternative treatments; and adapting to a healthy lifestyle that included a better balanced nutrition and the avoidance of unnecessary pressures. After about two months I began to feel an improvement. The frequent diarrhea stopped and my stomach was calmer. What didn't stop were the attacks of pain after certain meals and the vague feeling that the food was not being digested as it should be. The more the pains increased, the less I ate, and I lost weight and even the alternative therapists began to show signs of despair.

During one of those severe attacks, I took myself off to the emergency room at three in the morning. There, despite the steroids and the many other drugs that I received the pains did not recede for three hours. In the morning I was admitted to the department of internal medicine, where I met Dr R, who despite my stubbornness, succeeded in explaining to me the seriousness of my condition and the changes that were required, in her opinion, in the type of treatment. Until that meeting, I had for years avoided any kind of check-up at all regarding my disease. I had behaved like a small child who had been injured and because of the pain was afraid to show the wound.

It's possible that I was simply afraid of the tests themselves – most of them are not very pleasant to say the least – and I was afraid that they would only exacerbate my condition. Today, in retrospect, I can only thank Dr R who sat for a long hour in the middle of her working day to convince a stiff-necked (and -stomached) patient to do the tests.

For two weeks I was X-rayed from every possible direction, and at the end of it all a severe narrowing of the large intestine was discovered, which required an immediate operation, although, one of the other most important things they found from the tests was the relatively calm state of the inflammation. It seemed that two months of a calmer lifestyle and correct nutrition had done their job, However, the damage caused by active inflammation over an extended period could not be put right except with the help of an operation.

Every patient who believes he can continue living in a way opposed to the condition of his health should know and internalize that an active state of inflammation that continues for a long period causes permanent damage that sometimes is not immediately apparent. In my case the inflammation caused scarring on the walls of the bowel and the narrowing of one particular section of it. It was for that reason – and without any connection to my meal menu during that time – that an intestinal blockage could have occurred at any moment. This is what had caused the intense pains.

After receiving the results of all the tests and the recommendations of all the doctors, I was convinced. I was going to have the operation.

Under the knife

When I opened my eyes, it was to another world.

I had never had an operation, so I had no idea of what to expect. I had always thought that the preparatory procedures as well as the surgery itself would be the hard part. That was fiction. When I came round I was immediately struck by the strange sensation that this body stretched on the bed and connected to my head, was not the body I had known before I was anesthetized.

"What's the time?" was the first question. A quick calculation (and "quick" is a relative term) pointed to the fact that eight hours had gone by. Little by little I began to sense the poor state of my body, and I understood that the hard work still lay ahead of me. It was in fact only just beginning.

I recall the first night after the operation only vaguely. I was connected to four tubes at different places on my body. I was feeling very bad. The pain wasn't concentrated in any specific place. My entire body felt as if it had just been hit by a train speeding at 200 km an hour. I was lying on my back, but I couldn't move. I didn't even dream of stealing a glance at my stomach area out of fear of being exposed to the visual equivalent of the strange feelings that were emanating from there. About every two hours I asked for shots for the pain, which only seemed to have grown. In the morning, for a fraction of a second, I thought that everything had been a bad dream. However, the pains left no room for doubt – it wasn't a dream, it was a nightmare.

The intestine is a long tube whose role is to absorb the contents of the food[1], in my case, it was the stenosis (an area narrower than normal) that was preventing the food from passing through properly. The aim of the operation was to enable a smoother passage for the food all the way along the intestine. The surgery, which lasted for eight hours, included the removal of the part that connected the large and small intestines, known as the terminal ileum, and that contained the narrow bit, and the widening of yet other parts that were narrower than the normal. And all of this had been caused by the active inflammation.

The first days after the operation were extremely difficult. This was mainly as a result of the procedure of inflating the abdominal cavity, something that greatly interfered with my speaking and breathing for many days afterwards. Every slight movement in the bed was a painful reminder that not so long ago my internal organs had been reorganized. Still, the team of doctors from Surgery Ward B at Hillel Yaffe Hospital did not allow me to feel sorry for myself. Because they were concerned about pneumonia I was asked to get out of bed a few times a day. Because of the pain and my state of mind, I didn't really cooperate, but the moment that Dr A, the surgeon who had operated on me, part-threateningly told me that he would operate on me again if I didn't get up, I leapt from the bed within three seconds.

The days crawled by, and after the pessimism and shock in which I had been wallowing during the first few days, the pain began to fade. I felt that I could breathe more easily, and the amount of tubes that were connected to my body decreased.

---

[1] See Appendix: Anatomy of the digestive system

The operation

My unpleasant experiences continued, like the arrival one morning, between an infusion and injection, of the diagnosis of an infection in the operation wound – an infection that required a slight opening of the stitches (or, in the words of the surgeon: "it's going to hurt a little…"). A tip for life: when surgeons use the phrase "hurt a little", if you can, run!

During the recovery period, which was filled with experiences of the kind mentioned above, thinking was one of the only things I could do. I thought about the reasons that had brought me to this situation, about my lifestyle over the last few years, about all the things I had eaten although I had known I should not. I thought about the recklessness of not taking the disease into account when making decisions in my life.

About a week after the operation, I began eating again, and after another three days, I was discharged from the hospital. Those ten days of the recovery period had been the longest of my life. There is no doubt that without the support of my wife and my warm and loving family, overcoming this period would have been even harder, and for that I thank them from the bottom of my heart.

I will never forget those days in which I could not move from the bed – days in which every step to the toilet seemed an eternity, and every shower felt like a military operation. To this day memories of that time are an excellent incentive for me to take care of my body, so that at all costs I can avoid any similar experience in the future.

It is important to understand that as much as the operation repaired the damage in my case, there could be cases where a surgical solution cannot ease the damage done by the inflammation and all that it entails. Having said that, because I avoided doing some of the tests in time, I had been on the verge of requiring an emergency operation that would have been necessary had there been a complete blockage of the intestine. An operation like that requires a more serious opening of the stomach, with greater dangers and a longer period of recovery.

My operation resolved the specific problems caused by a state of active inflammation over an extended period. It is important to emphasize that its aim was not to heal the body of Crohn's disease. In most cases the disease is not content with just a part of the bowel, but appears in a number of places. It is sometimes liable to return, even after the affected area is cut out. The Crohn's patient should therefore never rely on surgical solutions, but should rather make use of other tools that will leave the disease in a state of inactivity.

So what do we do?

There are various ways to deal with the disease.

Disregard

"Yes, I have some sort of disease, but there's nothing that can be done about it"

The patient does not recognize his disease and continues his life out of a complete disregard for his limitations and medical condition. This method of dealing with it usually characterizes the period that comes after the discovery of the disease. It is accompanied by the (medical!) claim that says any preoccupation with the disease only encourages it, and precious energy should therefore not be wasted. This attitude simply betrays a lack of will to deal with reality. Because the patient is not prepared to recognize his disease, he does not change his lifestyle or his nutrition. The situation therefore quickly deteriorates, and the damage that follows the inflammation will not be slow in arriving.

War

"Crohn's is a disease like any other – doctor, give me pills!"

The patient assumes that because he was not born with the disease, it is separate from his body, and therefore it can be dealt with in the same way as with any alien entity that attacks the body – medication, and preferably strong medication. At the same time he neglects the repression of the various factors that encourage the disease, some of which are connected with lifestyle, nutrition, and others that have an influence on the spirit. The problem with this approach is that it ignores the fact that there is no wonder drug. The existing medication may succeed in repressing the inflammation (sometimes for extended periods), but will absolutely not succeed in repressing the disease.

Acceptance

"I'm a Crohn's patient, and the disease is an inseparable part of my body"

The patient (experienced, in most cases) is reconciled to the fact of his disease. He adapts himself to an appropriate lifestyle and recognizes the limitations that stem from the disease. This kind of behavior allows a lowering of the use of medication, and generally brings with it an improvement in the state of health. Because Crohn's disease is a psychosomatic illness (a physical illness that is influenced by psychological factors) it is very important to relate to the patient's psyche as an inseparable part of the factors that influence the disease. One of the negative outcomes that can be caused by patients' acceptance of the disease, is passivity in relation to its medical treatment. In extreme cases the patient is even liable to give up on conventional treatment, despite the fact that it can improve quality of life.

The truth, like everything in life, lies somewhere in the middle. Although we are not born with Crohn's or Colitis, they are still definitely diseases that require attention. The diseases are indeed an inseparable part of our bodies, and therefore we must relate to them, but having said that, there is no need to declare war on our bodies. In this war, as with most wars, there are only losers. If you'll allow me to be a little picturesque, the allegory of coping with the disease is one of climbing a smooth wet slope. The higher you get, the better you feel, and the struggle becomes easier. It's a pity, though, that the starting blocks are at the foot of the slope – the very point where the physical and mental feelings are difficult, belief in success is reduced, and the climbing is much more difficult.

At the start of the climb it's easy to stumble on the slippery ground, and to lose height. What is needed is skill, experience, patience and piles of motivation in order to maintain height and continue cautiously, inch by bowelled inch.

As a patient you can improve the way you cope with the disease with the help of various skills:

Gathering information

One of the important things that a Crohn's patient needs to do is to take decisions. These are difficult decisions, sometimes even fateful ones, and with the wrong decisions you are likely to pay a high price. Therefore, if your fate has been left in your hands, do your best to take decisions on the basis of as much information as you can get. Collect information from every source that comes to hand: talk to doctors and therapists, surf the web, gather information from books, learn from the experience of other patients, and of course from your own personal past experience (later I will show just how much of a central role personal experience plays in decision-making). Always remember that your own view comes before any doctor's opinion or therapist's recommendation, and that the weight of responsibility is on your own shoulders. If you decide wrongly, it is you who will pay the price. Gathering information is critical in avoiding a situation like this.

Knowing the tools

The 21st century offers Crohn's and Colitis patients a range of medications, both conventional and alternative. Medication – and I will expand on this later – is suited to various conditions, mainly with regard to their "intensity". While certain medications suit states of calmness in the disease, others are designed for situations in which hurricanes literally storm through your stomach. Using an unsuitable drug at the wrong time is liable to cause damage. Strong drugs are efficient in overcoming outbreaks of infection, but at the same time they are liable to inflict no small amount of damage on the body. Thus using them during times of quietness in the disease is to impose unnecessary danger. It is important to know the drugs thoroughly, their capacities and their suitability for dealing with the disease. And also, knowing the side-effects is no less important.

How to behave when the hurricane strikes

Firstly, it's important to quickly recognize that an attack is occurring in your body. You have to immediately reduce your amount of food, and to adjust its nutritional content to allow for easier digestion. At the next stage, after consultation with a doctor, you need to respond with drugs and therapies matching the kind of attack and the symptoms (diarrhea, pain, fever, etc.). At the same time it's important to maintain and take advantage of every ounce of energy with physical and mental rest, so that you can cope with the storm. (Sick leave from demanding work, or cancelling your participation in the triathlon would be a good idea.) The duration and strength of the attack determines the final bodily price you will pay in the future. You therefore need to use every tool you can find to help yourself. Neglect is criminal and reckless, especially during an attack.

How to behave when things are calm

Once the attack has passed, and a period of calmness arrives, the main thing is not to become complacent. You must continue gathering information, and learning the lessons from the last attack in order to try and avoid the next one. You must be sure to keep up your physical fitness, correct nutrition and a healthy lifestyle. On no account should you fall into the tempting traps of the modern world that offers bad nutrition, mental pressure and tiredness. Falling into these traps will only shorten the road to the next hurricane.

My way to a better life for the Crohn's and Colitis patient is made up of three parts (LMN):

Lifestyle

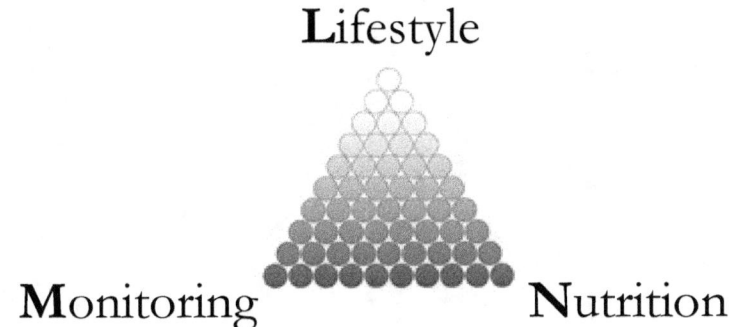

Monitoring   Nutrition

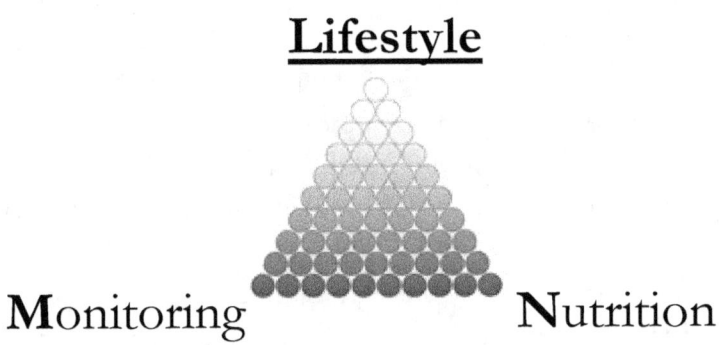

Lifestyle (LMN)

Any patient, wherever he is, can adopt a few rules that can meaningfully improve his physical and mental condition. Although some of these rules may seem simple and trivial, they are no less important than drugs or any kind or treatment. Their big advantage lies in their power to keep the patient in a stable physical condition and in their ability to avoid the struggle against a deterioration of the disease and against the side-effects of the drugs. These rules don't cost anything, but their effectiveness makes them priceless. They are the best way of attuning us to our body and its needs, and with their help we can learn how to succeed in the struggle together with our body, rather than being at war with it.

Learning the boundaries

In life we are expected to take many decisions on a variety of issues, from finding employment, a place to live, and choosing a partner, ordering a takeaway, or selecting a movie from a DVD library. For the average (and healthy!) reader some of these decisions are really important, and some are insignificant, but for Crohn's and Colitis patients, the most trivial of decisions can (and are likely to) have a direct effect on the body and the mind. The tiniest decisions (where should we eat lunch?) take on an extra significance, and therefore the bigger decisions (where should we work?) become crucial. As patients we have full responsibility for our health. We decide where we will eat, which medication to take, how many hours we sleep, and how to make a living. In order to do this it's important to learn, as far as possible, the limitations placed on us by the disease in every area of life, and we have to be careful not cross them. These limitations are dynamic, and change from time to time in accordance with the state of our health. Knowing one's limitations is not a simple matter for anyone, but it's important to recognize that in our case it's a way of fending off a deterioration in the disease. Crossing the borders will exact a price, while maintaining your framework will strengthen your health. Thus, the recommended lifestyle for Crohn's and Colitis patients includes lessening the pressure of the workplace, and ensuring that you eat in clean and hygienic places, something that would benefit the entire population. However, while a healthy person who isn't meticulous about this kind of lifestyle might bring increasing damage on himself over many years, the Crohn's or Colitis patient will pay an immediate and painful price.

Attack

The reasons for an attack

The character of the disease and its strength varies among patients and between various periods of time for any given patient. Accordingly, each patient can experience an attack in a different way. Having said that, the reasons for an extreme deterioration in the disease are similar for all patients:

- Consumption of low-quality food which stimulates the inflammation directly.

- Consumption of large quantities of high-fiber food that is hard to digest in large quantities (like fruit and vegetables). When food passes through the intestine its components rub against the bowel walls, and if these components are rich in fiber they can irritate sensitive areas of the bowel and cause pain that resembles that which arises from scratching and rubbing an open wound.

- Increased consumption of food that requires difficult and extended digestion (like meat).

- Consumption of large amounts of food within short periods of time, something that burdens the system and makes digestion difficult. What's more, if the inflammation causes narrowing in certain places in the bowel, food can accumulate and even get stuck. There is no need to tell you that this causes excruciating pain accompanied by noises and hardening of the stomach.

- If the inflammation is repeated, it can form scars on the bowel wall, and the narrowing can become permanent. If that happens the danger of attacks, even with the more careful consumption of food, is increased.

- In my personal experience, mental stress over an extended period can raise the danger of an attack. Our digestive system responds to our mental state, and when a person suffers from continued stress, vulnerable points will react accordingly. With Crohn's and Colitis patients the vulnerable point is the inflammation of the bowel.

What to do during an attack

When a person breaks his arm, it is splinted with plaster. The aim is to prevent certain movements that will hinder the proper knitting together of the break. During an attack our situation can be compared with that of the person who has broken his arm. Unlike that lucky person, the digestive system cannot be splinted with plaster. So we are left with the ability to endanger our digestive system. Therefore, in order to give the bowel the chance to heal properly, we need to make sure we follow the following rules:

- Avoid any unnecessary activity, we need to rest as much as possible, and to increase the amount of sleep we get.
- It's important to consult with a doctor as soon as you can, and to get help with medication as needed, even if you think you know what the doctor will have to say.
- Take advantage of alternative treatments that you have had experience with and have found to be effective.
- It's important to reduce your food intake because food irritates the digestive system and fuels the inflammation.
- You should not eat food that is difficult to digest like meat, vegetables and fried food.
- It's preferable to substitute solid foods with liquids (preferably soups that are not made from soup powder and that are seasoned as little as possible).
- It's important to increase your water intake and to reduce your consumption of natural juices that are rich in fiber. Also, drinking hot

herbal infusions that have a calming effect on the digestive system is recommended.

- You should grant as much rest to the digestive system and ease the digestive process as much as you can.

- It is hugely important to identify the attack early, and thus avoid any worsening of the situation. If it is not dealt with, the transition to a worsening of the attack itself will increase the chances of future attacks resulting from the damage done to the bowel.

- On the one hand it is important to allow the body to overcome the attack with its own resources. On the other hand, when the situation is serious, and is accompanied by symptoms such as a hard feeling in the stomach, excruciating pain, loud abdominal noises and high temperature, you must see a doctor immediately. This applies also in the case of pains and an inability to go to the bathroom – indications that there could be a blockage in the bowel.

- It is important to emphasize that although the natural tendency is not to eat during an attack, you should not take this too far. If the situation doesn't improve after a day's rest, you should not continue with your partial fasting, and you should be checked by a doctor. A situation in which the body lacks vitamins and liquids is very dangerous, and does not allow the body to fight the attack.

- Improvement in the severity of the inflammation is gradual and slow. In the difficult periods it is very easy to lose faith in your ability to return to a state of calm. It's important to remember, especially in those difficult moments that even the most stormy of hurricanes is temporary, and that it's always possible to improve the state of your health in order to keep the next hurricane at bay. Every small step in the right direction will bring you closer to that goal.

Taking advantage of the calm

"A common defect in human beings: during calm weather they do not take the storm into account..." Niccolo Machiavelli – *The Prince* [2] [i]

Crohn's disease and Colitis are characterized by extreme changes in the severity of the disease at different times. During periods when the disease is "calm" the patient appears to be healthy. He doesn't suffer from pains or frequent diarrhea, is able to eat anything and can in fact live his life without constraints. This is in contrast with other diseases such as celiac[3] and because of which the patient is not allowed to eat foods that contain gluten. Another is diabetes, which requires a continual balancing of sugar intake. There are no clear rules for Crohn's disease or Colitis, and the patient doesn't always know what he is allowed to eat, or how to behave. When the rules are not clear it's all the more difficult to follow them. This is especially true during periods when the patient is feeling good. It's at times like this, that the patient should not forget the difficult periods. It's exactly at these times that it's important to maintain correct nutrition and to strengthen the body with sporting activities.

---

[2] *The Prince* is a well-known philosophical book from the Renaissance period, written by Machiavelli about a prince who ruled Florence in the 16th century. The book consists of advice to the ruler on how to maintain and manage his rule, by means of, among other things, an analysis of the nature of man and an examination various historical issues.

[3] Celiac (or coeliac) is a medical condition arising from sensitivity to a protein called Gliadin, which together with another protein called Glutenin, comprise the gluten that is found in certain grains. For most people, the only treatment for all the symptoms (but which doesn't treat the disease) is the strict avoidance of foods that contain gluten – any food that contains wheat, barley or rye.

Only the experienced patient has felt in his own flesh just how correct the trite slogan is which proclaims "difficult in training, easy in battle". Along with strengthening the body it's important to be sure to do blood tests periodically in order to monitor the condition of the inflammation and to check whether the body's absorption of food is functioning well. It's very easy to be tempted to eat everything you desire, especially after the difficult periods of the disease when your diet is limited. However, every lapse like this is like an open invitation to the disease, which is just waiting for the right moment to stir up the hurricane inside us. The disease is always there. It doesn't disappear. It's what forces us, if you will – Crohn's and Colitis patients – to manage our lifestyles the right way.

In addition to this, continuing calm in the disease provides a good opportunity to turn towards the horizons of alternative treatments. Apart from their ability to strengthen the body and to improve the state of your health, they can also bring a reduction in your usage of medication – in agreement with your attending doctor, of course.

There are patients who succeed in recovering relatively easily from the bad times of the disease, something that is liable to cause them to be dismissive about their nutrition and their lifestyle. This phenomenon is typical mainly of young patients who stubbornly refuse "to give in" to the dictates of the disease. As one who was once a "young patient" I am very familiar with this attitude. During the first years I myself dealt with the disease in exactly the same way. Crohn's and Colitis have a lot of patience. At the end of the day they leave no choice to the arrogant patient but to acknowledge his limitations. The question is not whether it's going to happen, but when. The even more meaningful question is what price the patient will pay in the long term – a price exacted in the character, frequency and duration of the attacks. The more the patient maintains the disease in a state of remission, the more he will avoid complications and an aggravation of its intensity.

The journey to the toilet-bowl

One of the things that bothered me more than anything during the first years of my disease, was the fear of having to go to the bathroom outside of the house – either on a trip, or in any other public place. I was not at all afraid of an absence of bathrooms, but rather of the idea itself of visiting a toilet-bowl that I didn't know. As a boy, the very idea seemed to me unnatural an unacceptable. Years later I realized that there are people (also adults) who suffer from diarrhea and who fear going out of the house for long periods of time, only because of this unpleasantness. This experience is well-known to anyone who has found himself far from a bathroom with a sudden case of food-poisoning. For intestinal patients this is an almost daily reality. The vague feeling that begins to develop around the area of the belly-button, and with it the realization that something big is about to happen; the pressure that begins to spread after a few moments, accompanied by the fear that it will pass the point of no return before you can arrive at the coveted seat; the fear of the realization of "the doomsday scenario" only increases the activity of the digestive system that is already operating at full speed... by this stage you would give anything just to be alone at home with a bathroom that you have learned to know and love, and with no-one there to disturb your irritable bowel as it gives free rein to its needs.

Difficult matters indeed, friends.

There is, however, a very simple solution. It consists of two parts: the first – always, but always (not "usually" – but always!) keep toilet paper in your pocket, and in sufficient quantities. At the moment of truth, every square of it counts, especially where a sensitive digestive system is concerned, whose responses you can never know (you'll never succeed in understanding how that tiny cracker you ate can, in less than an hour, turn into the demolition of a building beneath you in the toilet bowl). The second component of the solution is the simple and consistent convincing of oneself that over time turns into an understanding that there is no, but no (I really mean it – no!) place where you cannot go to the bathroom. You will quickly discover that the realization that there is no need to run home every time you need to go is enough in itself to calm your system down.

Indeed, since I came by this wonderful knowledge, I have been invited less and less to my friends' houses, but the feeling of calm that accompanies me when I'm out of the house is worth the price.

Hygiene

One of the well-known complications of the disease is the development of hemorrhoids and various sores around the anus. The chances of this happening increase during periods when the disease is active, when the amount of daily bowel movements is larger. Accordingly, it is extremely important to be hygienic. It is important to ensure cleanliness in this sensitive area, with frequent washing as well as the use of wipes instead of toilet paper. The wipes reduce irritation and the chances of sores (and the environment and the environmentalists will please excuse me for this advice – I ask then to please take pity on the owners of sensitive bowels).

Sleep – allow the system to rest

It's hard to overstate the importance of sleep for patients who suffer from problems of the digestive system. It took me a long time to identify the connection between the state of my health and my sleeping habits. Today I am convinced beyond any doubt that a reduction in my hours of unbroken and restful sleep causes a distinct worsening in the state of my health – and vice versa: the more my body gets extended and better quality rest, the more the inflammation decreases and my body takes full advantage of the opportunity to heal itself. When it comes to sleep, it's important to ensure two things: quantity and quality.

The number of hours of sleep: The amount of sleep required differs from person to person. More than any medical research your own personal feeling as you wake up is a good enough tool to measure how much sleep you need. I strongly recommend that you try to sleep as much as you can – and definitely not less than six hours. Despite widespread public opinion to the contrary experts claim that the minimal required amount is eight hours a day. For me personally it's no less than seven hours, and I stick to that firmly (as much as my children will allow), and give up on most night-time activities (television is a disease for another book).

Quality of sleep: In order to give the body some real rest you need a deep level of sleep so that both body and soul are liberated and peaceful without any disturbance or external irritations. For most people it's the fifth phase of sleep, the dream phase, which comes only after a few hours of undisturbed sound sleep. Whoever suffers from stomach pains because of the disease definitely knows the difference between the feeling after a good night's sleep and the feeling after sleep that is of a lesser quality because of the pains. Be sure to get as much quality sleep as possible.

Some more recommendations relating to this:

- Avoid big meals for at least two hours before going to sleep. Eating before sleep causes activity in the digestive system during sleep, preventing it from resting. If you have to eat, eat things that are easy to digest, like yoghurt and soup.
- It's worth going to the bathroom before going to sleep, even if you don't really feel the need to – it cleanses and calms the system, allowing it to rest.
- Be sure to sleep in an environment that is as peaceful as possible so that you can get good quality sleep.

When the pains that accompany the disease are strong, they can continue during sleep, and thus influence both its duration and quality. As I've indicated, a lack of continuous quality sleep affects the seriousness of the disease, and hence also the intensity of the pains. What we have is a vicious circle, one of many that characterize the disease:

Pains ⟶ lack of sleep ⟶ worsening of the inflammation ⟶ pains.

In order to break the cycle there's sometimes no alternative to medication (with a doctor's approval) that eases the pain so that you can benefit from a deeper sleep that will help your body in coping with the disease.

Routine is not a bad thing

Because of the psychosomatic nature of diseases connected with the digestive system, it is recommended to be as calm as you can as much as you can. For most people times of change are characterized by a marked lack of calm accompanied by fears of the change. This is even more true of patients. There is a great danger of a deterioration during times like these. Changes can occur in any circumstances – in the workplace, at home, one's general lifestyle and so on. It's therefore very important to establish a permanent daily routine: It starts with your working hours and regular breaks, and ends with sporting activities, nutrition and sleeping habits.

It is well-known that life is not a picnic, and everyone has to deal with changes throughout life. However, it's possible to realize these changes in an enlightened way: When it comes to big changes it's important to plan accordingly so that our bodies and sprits will get through them smoothly. For example, in the case of moving to a different house you should ensure that you prepare all the arrangements well in advance so that the pressure points will be spread over a longer period and evaporate. More than that, the more stable your routine, the easier it is to include new elements in it in low doses, such as a new kind of food or sporting activity. In this way we can ease our bodies into accepting the dynamics imposed by our lives.

Health comes first

Here are some axioms that will help you to actualize this:

- There is no food that you absolutely have to eat. It's not important how much it costs, or how many long faces you might get.
- There is no workplace that cannot be replaced, and there is no situation for which there is no substitute.
- There is no day on which you cannot take a break.
- There is no activity that you cannot give up.
- There is no decision that does not first foremost take your health into consideration.
- The doctor or therapist is not God. When there is doubt, there is no doubt that you can always go to a different professional.
- There is no medication or treatment that you cannot stop. At the first sign of a problem, stop the treatment, in consultation with the doctor or therapist who prescribed it for you.
- There is no stomach ache that does not have a reason.
- Every person has an obligation to his health – everything else comes second.

Occupational therapy

The disease can impose a long period of enforced rest at home in order to allow the body to recover. So as not to be trapped in an inactivity that will bring boredom, which in turn brings on depression and restlessness, it's desirable to develop a hobby or two that will improve your feeling and turn your thoughts from negativity to positivity. Cooking, for example, is a good instance of something I have taken on. Take a book, download recipes from the internet, put on the apron (okay – you don't really have to) and fill the pots. After a couple of false starts, I assure you that something edible will come of it. Who knows – maybe you'll find a new career…Either way, you'll be able to enrich your menu with healthy dishes that you like, and with all the enjoyment of eating and preparation. For those of you who pass on the kitchen experience, try to find other areas of interest. The effort is worth the feeling that you have not given in to the disease. Even on bad days it's important to get out of bed, to do things, to feel creative (without disrupting your essential rest) and of course – to smile.

Physical activity

It's well known that physical activity is important for health, and this is all the more true for chronic diseases. You have to treat the coping with the disease as entirely a physical effort. Thus we can compare the effort our bodies invest in coping with the inflammation to the effort you invest in running. The more you practice, the better you will run, and the less effort it will require and the recovery time from the activity will be shortened accordingly. The body fights the disease in the same way. The better your level of physical fitness, the easier and more efficient the fight. Strengthen your body as much as it will allow. The results will not be long in coming.

It's important to remember that you need to match your sporting routine to the state of the disease. It's clear that during a period of activity in the disease, doing demanding physical activities is not recommended because it just exhausts the body and will sabotage its ability to recover. Having said that, it's worth taking advantage of the quiet periods to get the body into shape.

More than anything else, sport requires consistency. In order to keep up your motivation to maintain this consistency during the periods of change that the disease imposes, it's necessary to find the right sporting activity, one that brings enjoyment as well as satisfaction.

A comment on the subject of smoking

I don't smoke. I have enough problems. From conversations with patients who smoke, the evidence points to smoking causing a deterioration of the disease (beyond any other damage, of course). To Crohn's patients who smoke: If you're looking for another reason to stop – here it is. I am certain that the withdrawal from smoking is not an easy thing. Even so, during the course of a month, try to reduce your consumption of cigarettes by half, and see the change in the state of your health. In the case of Colitis it should be noted that research has shown that a return to smoking (however light) is likely to ease the symptoms of the disease, although this is only true for those patients who have smoked in the past.

Mental activity

As we've indicated, Crohn's, Colitis and other digestive diseases are psychosomatic diseases. From my personal experience, and from the experiences of others, I have no doubt that one's mental state has a direct influence on the state of the disease, without any connection to the way or the reasons the disease first appeared. For the doubters among you, try to go over in your minds and make out the connection between periods in which the disease deteriorated and those periods of stress in your life. I'm pretty certain that you'll be surprised to discover how strong the connection is.

The influence of the mind on the disease is a two-track one. It can improve things, but it can also cause a deterioration. A mental investment is therefore no less important than a physical one. What does this mean? First – identification. Just as you take note of the physical symptoms of the disease, you have to take note of the symptoms that are connected with your state of mind. This may not be an easy task, but with a little practice and routine it's possible. It's important to recognize signs of stress and depression already in the first stages in order to get rid of them as quickly as possible – whether by self-awareness and convincing, or with the help of your immediate circle, or by accepting professional help. Because of the nature of the disease it's very easy to find yourself in a cycle of stress that leads to a deterioration of the disease that in turn causes more stress. It's very hard to break this cycle on your own. Get help from family, friends and the experience of other patients (make use of the internet as a communications tool that allows you to share common experiences with other patients).

It's very natural and easy to ignore the pressures and stresses, and to relate only to the physical side of the disease. Don't give up! Once again, it's similar to the child we spoke about who held his wound tightly after falling, and refused to allow his parents or even himself to look at the site of the pain… Let go, look right into the pain, into the pressure and stress, and heal yourself. Be honest with yourself, and you'll be able to take advantage of the connection between mind and body in the fight against the disease. In this regard, I feel I have to give you a recommendation from the movies. The movie *What the Bleep is Going On?* or *Bleep* for short, flirting with modern physics, presents in the simplest way and from the most interesting angle, the potential of the influence of people on their bodies and their environment through thought.

There are various tools that help in treating and strengthening the mind. Different activities such as yoga and meditation provide particularly efficient tools for coping better with the disease and the obstacles it places before you. I'll speak more about Qigong[4] later, an ancient Chinese form of art based on movement and meditation. The chapter that deals with this was written by Dror Aloni a certified Qigong and Tai Chi[5] instructor, who struggled himself with a rare form of cancer. Apart from yoga and meditation, the abundance of possibilities among activities that strengthen the mind, are very diverse. Everyone can find the area that suits his character, beliefs and needs. Many patients invest great effort and money on the search for drugs for their disease, and are willing to travel great distances to find the expert who will be able to save them. One cannot of course put down medication and experts, but he who puts his faith in them alone is liable to lose all faith in finding other solutions that can be found within himself.

Dr Joseph Murphy in his book *The Power of Your Sub-Conscious Mind* [ii] provides a simple yet efficient approach, a theory which says that it is within the power of our thoughts to heal any disease.

"The source of all disease is in the mind. Nothing happens in the body unless there is some parallel and matched mental perception... there is only one healing process within people, and that is belief. There is only one healing power – the unconscious mind."

---

[4] Qigong or Ch'I kung: an ancient Chinese art of movement

[5] Tai Chi, or in its full name, Tai Chi Chuan, is a Chinese martial art originating from in the Kung Fu family

The general message of the book is that every thought, good or bad, that we think influences our sub-conscious, which is responsible for every bodily function, from its structure to its maintenance. Since every thought in our conscious mind also influences our sub-conscious, the final influence is on our bodies and health. It's important that we believe in our health and in our ability to heal ourselves. It is no less important to avoid negative thoughts that manifest themselves.

In Ekhart Tall's book *The Power of Now* [iii] he presents an approach according to which it's within our power to calm ourselves and to help our bodies by focusing on the present moment and surrendering to it. Many bodily tensions are caused as a direct result of stress and the continuous activity of thought. A number of techniques are presented in this book that help in bringing calm and relief from pressure by focusing on the present moment.

"The key is to be in a state of continual connection with your inner body – to feel it all the time. If your attention is attuned to your body as much as possible, you will be anchored in the moment. You will not lose yourself in the external world. And you will not lose yourself within your own head. Be focused on your body and on what you are doing in that moment..."

"Don't focus on a hundred things that you will do, or will need to do at any time in the future, but just on the one thing that you can do now. Be sure that you are not screening movies in your head and projecting yourself into the future thereby losing the moment."

I have no doubt that our minds have a direct influence on the state of our health. It would be silly to disregard as meaningless tools of this kind. These are tools that do not demand a great effort. They do not have any side-effects, and all that is needed to actualize them is a little belief.

Make no mistake – although most of the material that deals with calming the spirit is philosophical in one way or another and can't be digested by everybody (especially not by people with digestive problems). I found a more practical approach in the book *Manual of Freediving* [iv] . Freediving is a form of diving in which no breathing equipment is used. The longer a diver can hold his breath, the deeper he can dive. The book describes yoga and meditation techniques that help one to reach a physical calmness that heals the muscles in the body together with a mental serenity that calms both spirit and thought. These techniques have been proven to enable free divers to do this as a result of slowing the metabolism, reducing the heart-rate and the minimizing the cost of physical activity. The record for freediving today stands at a depth of about 214 meters and remaining underwater for over nine minutes. (Don't try this at home).

The techniques that help the free diver include, among other things yoga exercises that concentrate on breathing, meditation with the aid of guided imagery. These techniques can help Crohn's and Colitis patients, among other things to cope better with the disease by calming the pressures that accumulate in one's daily life.

I heartily recommend to every patient who is interested in recovering not to disregard experimenting with these tools that have to do with the mind. I don't mean this only for the spiritual among us, but also and especially for those of little belief, who regard the matter with doubt and cynicism. As one who was once counted among the doubters, no-one knows as much as I do that this change in my thoughts was not at all simple. It requires no little effort to experiment truthfully with the aid of these tools. And I'm sure that you will agree with me that cynicism never helps. You don't have to become a Buddhist monk. You can begin in a small way, with measured steps, by introducing calming exercises that will balance the intense activities of real life. In this way, with time, it is possible to arrive at a deep and positive change in your thought processes that can contribute in a real way to an improvement in the state of your health.

"I believe that a simple and unpretentious life is good for every person and is beneficial for the body and the soul..."
Albert Einstein – *Ideas and Opinions* [v].

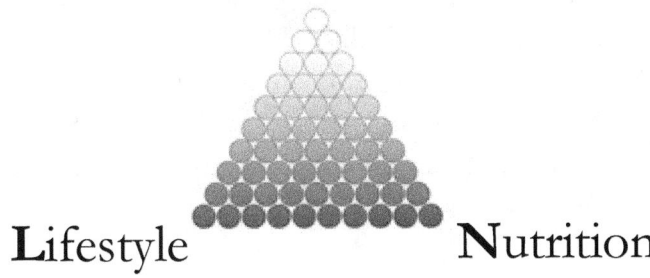

Monitoring

Lifestyle   Nutrition

Monitoring and Treatment (LMn)

There is currently no cure for Crohn's and Colitis. Existing drugs can only suppress them. All drug-based treatments impact patients differently, according to the level of the disease. This vagueness complicates the treatment. It's happened more than once that patients have had to take it on themselves to make decisions (in consultation with the doctor) that have a direct influence on their condition. Taking the correct decision requires knowledge concerning the nature of the treatment or test, and being well-informed on all the parameters that contribute to the patient's bodily and mental state over a long period.

The patient who is forced to devote most of his strength to deal with the disease needs to enlist additional energy for tests and treatments. An understanding of the aim of the test and treatment tends to increase the motivation to undergo them. For every patient, choosing a suitable treatment is based on being well-informed about its aim, as well as on frequent monitoring of the situation.

This chapter investigates treatment methods and monitoring for both Crohn's and Colitis, methods that include medical and self-monitoring systems, and conventional and alternative approaches to treatment. The aim of the chapter is to provide information to patients that will aid them in taking decisions concerning how they should monitor their disease and methods of treating it.

The art of monitoring

Crohn's and Colitis are characterized by variability in the seriousness of the inflammation. This variability is influenced by many parameters that change all the time. The only way you can sense most of these changes is by periodic testing.

The monitoring needs to include tests of the patient's general health, and not to focus only on the inflammation itself. This is because of the influence of the disease on general health and vice-versa.

In this chapter I will detail the different methods of monitoring our state of health, and I will show how the patient himself can contribute to completing the full picture with the help of self-monitoring of different parameters. An explanation of how to interpret blood tests and a presentation of the various conventional tests will round off the subject. It's preferable for the patient to acquire a knowledge of the range of monitoring methods, the various tests and their aims for himself, so that when the time comes he won't be afraid of them, and will be able to choose the right type of test, and the most suitable time to do it.

"If you know your enemy and you know yourself you will not be hurt in a hundred battles; if you don't know your enemy, but you do know yourself, you will win some and lose some; if you don't know your enemy and also do not know yourself, you will be hurt in every battle..."

Sun Tsu, *The Art of War* [6] [vi]

Self-monitoring

In contrast with all the tests that the patient is compelled to do, self-monitoring is not likely to bring about any worsening of the inflammation or general state of health, and it doesn't include invasive tests. Monitoring is important in that it can help the patient to understand his special needs, to assist him in completing the picture of the state of his health and sometimes even to avoid the need for tests that involve danger.

The aim of monitoring

The aim of monitoring is to collect data about the disease. From the accumulated data it's possible to answer a number of key questions:

- How is the disease affected by the various drugs that the patient is consuming?
- What is the effect of the different alternative treatments on the disease?
- What is the role of the patient's state of mind – in particular his mood?
- What is the effect of nutrition on the disease, and which foods aggravate or improve the patient's medical condition?

---

[6] The book *The Art of War* by Sun Tsu was probably written in the 3rd century BCE. It is known as one of the most influential books on military strategy, and even today still has an influence on other fields connected with implementing strategy and taking decisions.

- Does the patient's daily routine and changes to it, affect his medical condition?

Tools for monitoring

Collecting data can be accomplished in a number of ways, from the Excel program to drawing up tables on a sheet of paper. In my view, it is very important to write down every tiny detail, at least in the initial stages of monitoring. Only after you have recorded your daily life in numbers and dry data, will you be able to draw conclusions regarding your nutrition and lifestyle. Even if you don't like accountants, you have to agree with them that it's hard to argue with numbers. Thus, facts that you were not prepared to admit, or that you have succeeded in distorting, will suddenly shout out from your table and will force you to acknowledge reality, and to make the necessary changes.

You need motivation for monitoring, and ensure that you're honest and that you pay attention to detail. It's important to be objective and not judgmental. In that way you'll be able to collect exact data and draw conclusions that will serve you well later on.

An example of periodic monitoring

The data presented in this paragraph is the result of some self-monitoring that I did over about six months in 2005. With the aid of this data I came to important conclusions that serve me to this day. It is a daily monitoring that is suitable for a period of a number of months. All the information is concentrated on one Excel spreadsheet, and produces a general picture of changes that occurred during that period. For convenience I'll present it separately in sections of nine days for each category.

Data representing the state of my health and general sensitivity:

Date	Daily bowel movements	Weight	A lot of pain = 10 Pain	Feeling great = 10 Feeling very bad = 0 General feeling
29 Apr 05	4	62	6	4
30 Apr 05	6	62	4	3
01 May 05	4	62	4	4
02 May 05	3	62	3	5
03 May 05	2	62	1	6
04 May 05	2	62	1	6
05 May 05	1	62	1	6
06 May 05	1	62	1	7
07 May 05	1	62	0	8

- "Daily bowel movements" – The amount of bowel movements is usually in direct proportion to the severity of the inflammation.
- "Weight" – An important parameter. Embodies the amount of food needed and its absorption by the body. Also, a loss of weight tends to suggest diarrhea. Desired weight varies for individuals according to their age, height and sex.
- "Pain" – indicates the level of pain I experienced, if at all, on the day. The level of pain is of course subjective, although the results are measured in relation to the patient so that they can provide an indication of changes in this parameter.
- "General feeling" – Indicates general health. A parameter that in fact summarizes my feelings on the day.

From this data it is very clear that on Saturday 30 April 2005 I suffered an attack accompanied by pain and diarrhea, an attack that lessened in severity as the week progressed. As I will show in a moment making a simple comparison of this data with the data that appears in the following paragraphs, it's possible to estimate in a fairly accurate and clear way, the amount of influence of one aspect on another.

Medication and Alternative treatments appear in the following table:

	3 mg	0.5 g	Herbal remedies			
Date	Budesone	Pentasa	Pills	Infusion	Tincture	Chamomile
29 Apr	2	4	3	1	2	0
30 Apr	3	4	3	0	1	2
01 May	3	4	3	1	3	2
02 May	3	4	3	2	3	2
03 May	3	4	3	1	2	0
04 May	3	4	3	1	2	0
05 May	3	4	3	1	1	0
06 May	3	4	3	0	2	0
07 May	2	4	3	1	2	0

At that time my treatment included various doses of Pentasa[7] and Budesone[8] (steroids). The data in the table present the amount of pills per day that I consumed every day. At the same time I was getting herbal remedies that included the drinking of a tincture[9] (a liquid that concentrates plants with the aid of alcohol). The infusion and the pills consist of powder that is produced from plants. On

---

[7] Pentasa: www.drugs.com/pentasa.html

[8] Budesonide: www.drugs.com/mtm/budesonide.html

[9] Tincture: An extraction in alcohol of a medication that is produced from a plant

Saturday 30 April 2005 I increased the dosage of steroids during the attack and I drank more chamomile. As we have seen in the table in paragraph 1, following this, the attack lessened in intensity. The fact of my recording of the substances that I consumed and the minimal combination of steroids and herbs helped me to overcome the attack, and assisted me in dealing with future attacks.

Daily nutritional data:

Date	Day	Max. 10 Daily amount of food	Eggs	None = 0 Lots = 5 Grains and pulses	Bread and pasta
29 Apr	Fri	3	2	0	0
30 Apr	Sat	2	2	0	1
01 May	Sun	1	2	0	0
02 May	Mon	2	2	1	2
03 May	Tues	3	2	1	2
04 May	Wed	3	2	1	2
05 May	Thurs	3	2	1	2
06 May	Fri	3	2	0	2
07 May	Sat	5	2	3	2

Date	Milk	Chicken/Meat	Fish	Veg/Fruit	Veg Juice
		None = 0 Lots = 5			
29 Apr	0	0	0	0	1
30 Apr	0	0	0	0	0
01 May	0	0	0	0	0
02 May	0	0	0	0	0
03 May	0	0	0	0	0
04 May	0	0	0	1	0
05 May	0	0	0	1	0
06 May	1	1	0	0	0
07 May	0	2	0	1	0

This table records data concerning my nutrition. With the help of this data I was able to locate and isolate food products that caused a deterioration in the inflammation, and other products that helped in suppressing it.

"Daily amount of food" – The primary aim of this data is to confirm that I don't eat less than necessary. The measurement is personal, where the rating 5 represents the recommended amount for a person of my age and height. It is recommended that you consult with a dietician who specializes in the daily menu for diseases of the bowel. As I have indicated, the disease can cause a suppression of the appetite, and one can therefore not overstate the importance of this measurement. One should not overdo a reduction in the amount of food and it's importance to continue supplying the body with the intake it needs.

It can be seen that during the attack I reduced the amount of food to the minimum, almost no vegetables and meat. After a week my body recovered from the attack, and I returned to eating chicken.

Various daily activities, components of stress, and daily summary:

Date	Day	Hours of sleep	Max = 10 Fitness	Stressed= 10 Feelings of stress	Excellent = 10 Daily summary
29 Apr	Fri	12	4	5	5
30 Apr	Sat	8	0	6	3
01 May	Sun	9	0	3	2
02 May	Mon	9	1	2	4
03 May	Tues	7	1	2	6
04 May	Wed	7	0	2	5
05 May	Thurs	7	0	2	6
06 May	Fri	9	1	0	6
07 May	Sat	8	5	0	7

Date	Day	Main activity	Comments
29 Apr	Fri	Studies at home	Haven't felt well for a few days
30 Apr	Sat	Studies at home	Attack of pain and diarrhea
01 May	Sun	Rest	Day of recovery, soup and 2 eggs, less pain
02 May	Mon	Studies at home	Studies, soup without powder and rice.
03 May	Tues	Studies	Studies, soup, rice, sandwich with hard-boiled eggs
04 May	Wed	Studies	Studies, soup, rice, sandwich with hard-boiled eggs
05 May	Thurs	Studies	Studies, sandwich, eggs and rice.
06 May	Fri	Studies at home	Day of study at home, eggs, a little home-made pizza, chicken
07 May	Sat	Sea	Sea, chicken, potato, eggs, bread, soup

"Hours of sleep" – This indicates the amount of sleep during the night before the indicated day. I recommend writing it down like this in order to check its influence on the situation during the day.

Monitoring this parameter clarified for me in an undeniable way how important sleep is in the struggle to deal with the disease. What is clearly impressive in this example is how the many hours of sleep I managed to get since the beginning of the attack, played an important part in my recovery.

"Fitness" – This indicator helps in maintaining stability and consistency in sporting activity during calm periods.

"Feelings of stress" – This is perhaps the most surprising parameter in terms of its relationship to the state of the disease. The monitoring I did during my studies clearly indicates that the mental stress causes a deterioration in the disease. It's possible to see in this example that on the day I had the acute attack I experienced a relatively high level of stress. Amazingly, similar events also occurred during the following months and fully confirmed my conclusion.

"Daily summary" – This indicator sums up my feelings on the day: Did I manage to do everything I wanted to? Did I have the strength and desire to do various things during the day, and so on. I decided to include this indicator in order to get a more accurate picture of my feelings on the day, feelings that have an influence on the disease.

"Main activity" – This indicates the main thing I did during the day: work, study, rest entertainment and so on. In this way I could connect particular activities to deterioration or improvement in my condition, and even to find additional connections like that between mental stress and particular activities during the day.

In the "Comments" column I have included additional details that don't fit within the other parameters, but seem to have a potential importance in reaching future conclusions.

Analysis of the data

From the wide range of connections and conclusions that one can draw from the data, I have chosen to present a number of key examples:

- The comparison between the general feeling and the level of mental stress that I felt on those particular days:

    (The data relates to the excellent period described in the previous paragraphs.)

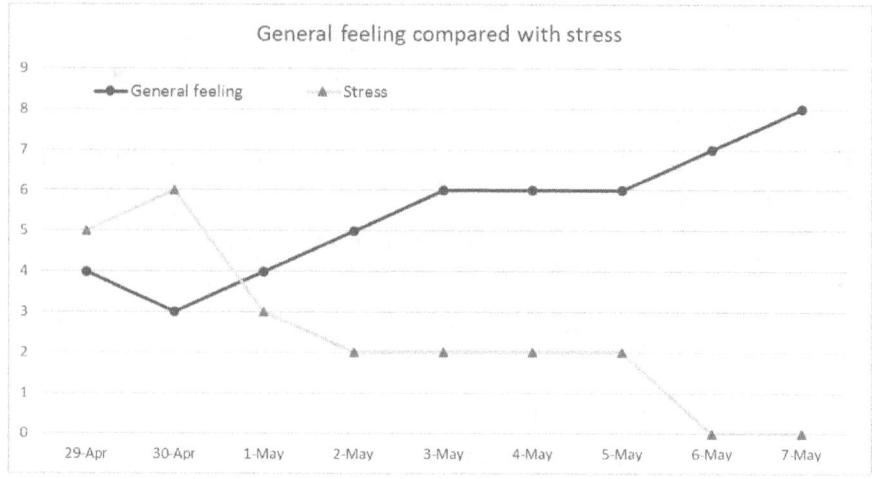

The inverse relationship (negative correlation) between the general feeling, which includes the state of my health, and the level of stress is clearly demonstrated here.

- The daily consumption of meat or chicken in relation to the pain I experienced on the day:

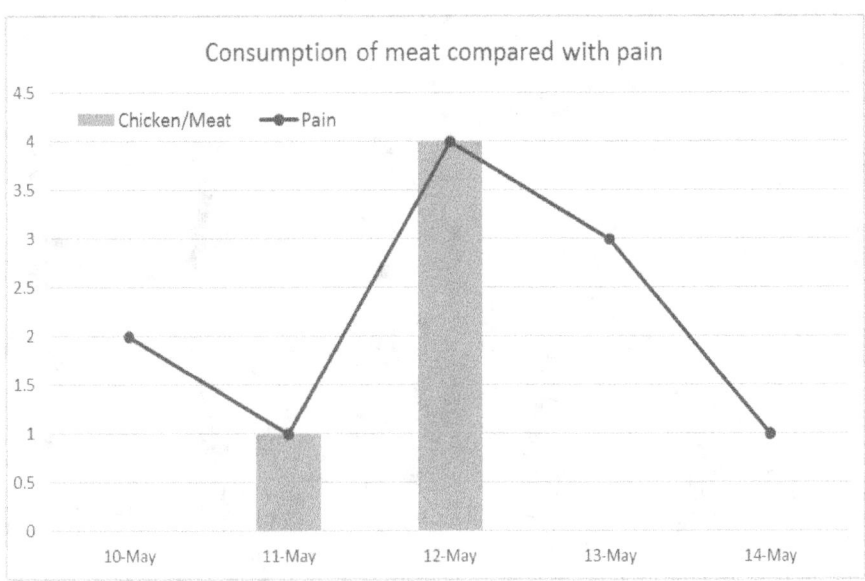

From this data, repeated in other cases, it was clear to me that meat is indeed difficult to digest, and is liable to cause pain.

- The influence of herbal remedies:

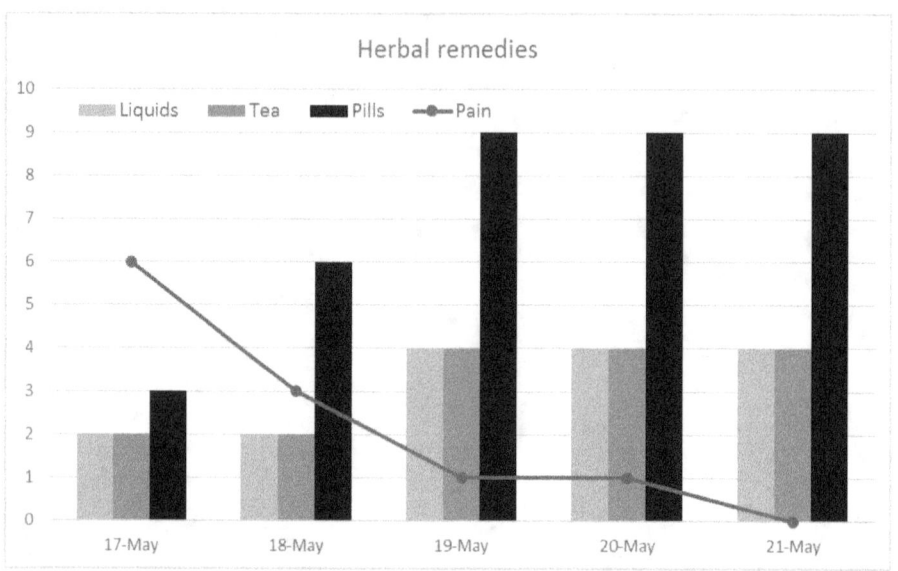

In my experience, the influence of alternative herbal remedies requires longer periods of monitoring and isolation of the treatment, in order to be able to draw conclusions about the effectiveness of the treatment. Despite the difficulty it's definitely desirable to monitor all alternative treatment (and at the same time, also conventional treatment, of course) and to become aware of its effectiveness.

Naturally the results of the monitoring I presented here are valid only for myself, but the method of managing the monitoring and drawing conclusions, can be useful for any patient.

The data cited above gives just a taste of the benefits that one can obtain from detailed, honest and quality monitoring.

For more on this please see Appendix 3 – Index of the seriousness of the disease: Crohn's Disease Active Index (CDAI).

An example of monitoring the eating of problematic foods

I am going to monitor every food that causes stomach pains by means of rating it on the "5-Bang Scale".

A food that scores 5 points is considered a problematic food and one should minimize its consumption as much as possible.

For example, products made from cow's milk and hot seasoning would be identified as problematic foods on this table:

Food	1	2	3	4	5
Eggs	X				
Chicken	X	X			
Beef	X	X	X		
Fish	X				
Fresh Veg	X	X			
Cooked Veg	X				
Cow's milk products	X	X	X	X	X
Goat milk product	X				
Potato	X	X			
Fried food	X	X	X	X	
Hot seasoning	X	X	X	X	X

Instructions for constructing the list:

- Every new food that causes discomfort should be added to the list.
- You should fill in the table on the basis of your personal experience and not according to the recommendations of others.
- Only place foods that were the main part of the last meal on the list, for example for a meal in which you have eaten a mainly beef and only a little rice, you should mark down the beef. In order to improve the ability to identify problematic foods it is worth planning more meals that include only one type of food. For example eat only rice or pasta in one meal, and monitor your stomach's response.
- Do not include foods that you do not eat at home (such as you might eat in restaurants and cafeterias) because you will not be able to monitor the quality of the food.
- Only add a food to the list if you feel bad from it; if you felt bad already before the eating the food, don't mark it down on the list.
- You should wait a week between two ratings of the same food
- Don't mark down identical foods. If, for example, you felt bad after eating fried potato, your next rating should be for baked or roast potato. Thus, if you felt bad after eating chicken with fresh vegetables your next rating should be only for chicken in a meal that does not include fresh vegetables. In this way you can isolate the problematic components.
- You should include the manner of cooking or seasoning. For example, fried meat patties require ratings in the categories of beef and fried food; chicken wings in a hot sauce require ratings in the chicken and hot seasoning categories.
- You should mark your ratings down only during periods of routine. For example, if you are going through a period of stress in your life, or if you are not sleeping enough, you should not mark ratings because you will not be able to isolate the real causes of your discomfort.

An example of a list of common foods:

Food	1	2	3	4	5
Eggs					
Chicken					
Beef					
Fish					
Fresh Vegetables					
Cooked Vegetables					
Fruit					
Cow's milk products					
Goat's milk products					
Rice					
Pasta					
White bread					
Whole wheat bread					
Snacks and nuts					
Sweets					
Fried food					
Hot seasoning					
Powdered or ready foods					
Carbonated drinks					
Coffee					
Tea					

The list is of course not a final one and you can always add new foods.

You can increase the level of detail: for example, you can break down the entry for vegetables into tomatoes, cucumbers, carrots and so on.

An example of monitoring over an extended period

During the years with the aid of these tools I have learned my body's responses to nutrition and lifestyle changes. In addition it was important for me to maintain the monitoring of the different treatments and the state of my health over an extended period so that I could get a general picture and to draw conclusions that would improve the state of my health.

I arrange my monitoring in an Excel spreadsheet (but you can do it in any way you choose). Every event connected to the state of my health appears in a new line so that I have a diary that describes events with the dates on which they occurred. An even might be the start of a new conventional or alternative treatment (or changes in dosage), a change for the better or the worse in the state of my health, getting back test results, the appearance of new symptoms, or a change in lifestyle – anything that is important to you. This diary can work for self-monitoring, and is useful for visits to the doctor who is treating so that you can go over when you started your medication and what worked better in the past.

The entries that I update for every event are: the amount of bowel movements per day, weight, general feeling, level of stress at the time, quality of sleep and data received from blood tests: CRP (the level of inflammation active in the body) and the level of iron (important for proper functioning of the body). In addition to this I describe changes, nutrition and bodily functions, and I indicate starts or pauses of medication courses.

I describe every event and general feeling, draw conclusions if there are any, and mark down what works, and what doesn't. For example, I discovered that a certain type of antibiotic is not effective for me, or that at a certain point I could eat bananas without incident and found that they helped in stopping diarrhea.

An example documenting three events:
(with a presentation of some of the data)

Date	Imuran 50 mg	Nutrition	CRP	Good = 10 General Feeling	Condition
26 Mar			0	8	Yellow
03 Feb	Start x 2 per day	Stop chicken, begin fish only	-	5	Orange
20 Jan			22	3	Red

In the first event in January (20 Jan 05) I didn't feel well (General Feeling 3) and obtained blood test results: CRP = 22

In the second event in February (03 Feb 12) I felt a little better. I began to take Imuran 50 mg, and I effected a change in nutrition, which included substituting chicken for fish as the main component of my daily menu.

In the third event in March (26 Mar 12), I felt better (General Feeling 8) and obtained blood test results: CPR = 0, confirming a lowering of the level of inflammation in the body.

Each event includes a description of the condition represented by a color. The following is an explanation of the five different conditions:

Condition Red

- Description of the condition: A difficult period accompanied by attacks, or after an attack accompanied by diarrhea or pain.
- Activities for this condition: Increase rest, stop physical activities, reduce activities outside the home and consult with the attending doctor regarding treatment for the attack – for example, antibiotics.
- Nutrition for this period: Mainly liquids, real chicken soup without powder, tea infusions, a little goats-milk yoghurt with honey, soft-boiled eggs, and drinking plenty of water.

Condition Orange

- Description of the condition: A relatively low level of pain or diarrhea.
- Activities for this condition: Increased rest, reduced and relaxed physical activity that calms the body and spirit.
- Nutrition for this period: Increase liquids, and only a little solids – mainly cooked vegetables.

Condition Yellow

- Description of the condition: Feeling well but not stable.
- Activities for this condition: Be careful with nutrition and increase rest. Return gradually to normal physical activity.
- Nutrition for this period: Solids, but take care with fruit and vegetables. Try a few bananas, dates and vegetable and fruit juices, well-strained and without the peels.

Condition Blue

- Description of the condition: Feeling well without pain or diarrhea – stable for more than a month.
- Activities for this condition: Increase physical activity, continue with good rest at night and good nutrition.
- Nutrition for this condition: Eat foods that are known not to be problematic. Try a little fruit and vegetables without the peels.

Condition Green

- Description of the condition: Feeling well for an extended period – more than six months.
- Activities for this condition: Enjoy life, increase physical activity and try to increase weight.
- Nutrition for this period: Maintain quality nutrition, also – you can try out new foods with care, and monitor the response.

Blood tests

Blood tests are one of the efficient and less painful ways of monitoring your health. Blood is involved in almost every process that happens in the body. Among other things, it is responsible for the conveying of oxygen and other substances to every part of the body, and therefore for cleansing the body of waste. As you know, blood tests are among the simplest tests that a patient is required to undergo, even more so for a bowel disease patient. The test is done by means of blood samples taken from the patient's body and sent to a laboratory for testing. There the blood constituents are analyzed, and the patient's functioning and state of health are diagnosed.

From the vast range of measurements that can be generated from blood samples I will obviously focus on those that relate to bowel disease, among them the CRP and ESR tests which provide indications of active inflammation in the body, and the level of vitamin B12 and iron, the lack of which is liable to cause tiredness and weakness (something that a bowel disease patient cannot afford).

You will find a description of the tests and their meaning in Appendix 2. The data is intended only to broaden your knowledge, and are of course is not a substitute for a diagnosis by your doctor. As I have previously noted, knowledge is power, especially in the light of the special characteristics of the disease, and the need to take decisions.

Anemia [10]

Anemia is a condition in which a person suffers from a low level of hemoglobin or a lack of red blood cells. Hemoglobin is a protein found in red blood cells, and its main function is to carry oxygen from the lungs to the various organs of the body.

The causes of anemia are lack of iron, faulty production of hemoglobin, lack of vitamin B12 or folic acid, bleeding and more. These causes can stem from chronic illness – especially of the digestive system – that impact on the good absorption of vitamins.

The symptoms stem first and foremost from a lack of oxygen in the organs, something that causes paleness, weakness, tiredness, dizziness, headaches and so on. More than that, the body activates a number of compensatory mechanisms in order to oxygenate the tissue, among them raising the heart and respiratory rate.

Treatment is matched to the type of anemia. Lack of iron, vitamin B12 or folic acid is treated by enriching daily food consumption with these ingredients alongside the taking of supplements.

If the anemia is caused by bleeding, the bleeding must be stopped. With chronic diseases of the digestive system it is particularly important to pay attention to any lack of these vitamins, a lack that causes exhaustion and impairs the ability to deal with the disease. It is therefore important, in accordance with a doctor's instructions, to undergo periodic monitoring by means of blood tests.

---

[10] John W. Adamson. The Anemia of Inflammation/Malignancy: Mechanisms and Management
asheducationbook.hematologylibrary.org/cgi/content/full/2008/1/159

Sometimes, even after changing your menu or adding supplements, the results do not change. This is mainly because of a lack of absorption of vitamins in the body. When this happens the doctor is likely to recommend injections, or vitamin transfusions directly into the circulation.

* There are other types of anemia that stem from other diseases, and which are not relevant here.

Conventional medicine -
Treatment methods and monitoring

"Time thrusts everything before it and can bring with it the good as well as the bad, and the bad as well as the good... If the problem is not dealt with: war cannot be prevented, only postponed..."

Niccolo Machiavelli – *The Prince* [i]

In order to understand how western medicine deals with Crohn's disease, I interviewed Prof Zvi Fireman. Prof Fireman is the Director of the Institute of Gastroenterology (diseases of the digestive system and liver) at Hillel Yaffe Medical Center. In the course of his work, Prof Fireman has been treating Crohn's and Colitis patients for more than twenty years. Other sources for this chapter include various articles appearing in the professional literature and on the internet. It is my intention to present here a summary of the general information concerning conventional medical treatments. There is too little space here to deal with the subject in full. Thus, if you wish to complete your knowledge about it, I recommend that you take medical advice and consult official sources like medication inserts, about which I will speak later. In addition, you can also refer to Appendix 1 – Anatomy of the Digestive System, which clarifies the names of the various organs of the digestive system that also appear in this chapter. You should consult with your doctor with regard to any drug treatment.

Definition

Inflammatory Bowel Disease (IBD):
An inclusive name for inflammatory diseases of the digestive system, of which the main ones are Crohn's and Colitis.

Crohn's disease (CD):
A chronic disease that affects the digestive system and which can appear along the entire length of the system – from the mouth to the anus. The areas most susceptible to the disease:

- The terminal part of the small intestine – the point of connection between the small and the large intestine, also known as the Terminal Ileum.
- The large intestine (appears in half of the cases together with impairment to the small intestine).

Ulcerative Colitis (UC):
A chronic inflammation that appears only in the large intestine and the rectum. With Colitis the inflammation is continuous and involves only the mucus. It does not penetrate the entire intestinal wall. The reasons for the disease, and its identification and treatment, are similar for the two diseases, despite the clinical differences between them.

Crohn's and Colitis are diseases that have a stronger effect on the immune system which then displays uncontrolled activity, in all likelihood against the germs that are found in the bowel. The reasons for the appearance of the disease are not known. There a few theories such as a disturbance of the immune system, a bacterial or viral infection, hereditary disease, psychosomatic reasons, poisoning, damage, and so on. The reason is probably based on a combination of genetic background and environmental factors of the kind I have mentioned. Currently it is not possible exactly pinpoint the factors and therefore it is not possible to prevent the disease from appearing.

About twenty years ago, throughout the world, the disease was found mostly among Jews, but in recent years a similar percentage of non-Jews have been found to have the disease. Although the connection has not been proven in the research, it's possible to tell from this that it has occurred along with the socio-economic improvement of these populations.

The disease is equally common to men and women, and can appear at any age. In most cases it breaks out at the end of the second decade of life (between the ages of sixteen and twenty) and is connected to a stressful period of the patient's life (for example, army service).

An estimation of the number of patients

The frequency of Crohn's disease is between ten and seventy patients for every 100,000 of the general population. (It more frequent among Jews of the diaspora).

Unofficial research points to an increase in the number of Crohn's and Colitis patients globally in recent years.

Symptoms of the disease

- Chronic diarrhea: One of the most prominent symptoms of the disease. It can appear without warning and continue for long periods. It is usually accompanied by strong odors and even bleeding.
- Pain: Stomach pains caused by intestinal cramps are the main and most prominent and common symptoms of the disease. The pains usually begin on the lower right side of the abdomen. The pains vary from general discomfort to acute stomach pains with strong cramping of the intestines.
- Temperature: Intense activity in the disease – especially in severe cases – includes the development of fistulae (a connection between tissues – please see the explanation later on), or ulcers – accompanied by high temperature and shivers.
- During later stages it is possible to note other symptoms such as: Weight loss, signs of malnutrition, anemia, lack of appetite and lack of vitamins. In addition, following continuous diarrhea, damage to the anus can occur, and also injury to other systems and tissues such as joints, skin, eyes and liver.
- Blood in stool: Characteristic of Colitis, blood mixed with feces can occur with the involvement of the large intestine. Fresh blood is a generally a sign of the involvement of the rectum.
- A continual need to move the bowels, or tenesmus: Characteristic of Colitis, in which the patient can feel a continuous need to go to the bathroom, but without result, or with a mucous discharge only.

The clinical expression of the disease varies from patient to patient. There are patients who suffer from an isolated attack that closely resembles inflammation of the appendix, and enjoy a full recovery after a successful treatment with medication. In contrast to them there are patients who suffer from the harshest aspects of the disease – high-frequency severe attacks including even symptoms outside of the intestine such as fistulae, or narrowing of the intestine. This group is characterized by rises and falls in the activity of the inflammation, but for most it will never disappear. In recent years there have been attempts to create all kinds of medical parameters to characterize the disease and the level of its severity. So far none of these attempts have been successful.

Possible complications of the disease (not for anyone with a weak heart)

Fistula – An abnormal connection between tissues (between two internal organs or between an organ and an area on the surface of the body). For example, a connection between the intestine and the bladder, or in women, the pelvic floor or the vagina. These connections are caused by the active inflammation of the outer wall of the intestine, and are liable to cause infection and various complications. A typical complication among Crohn's patients.

Narrowing of the intestine – The intestine is a kind of flexible tube. If it is narrower than normal in one particular area it does not allow the normal passage of food. This can cause severe problems in digestive functioning, vomiting, pain in the narrow area and a rise in temperature. The narrowing is a result of the inflammatory process, and includes swelling and scarring of the intestinal wall. A typical complication among Crohn's patients.

Blockage of the bowel – This occurs in the narrow area when the intestinal walls stick together. This condition does not allow the passage of food at all, and requires immediate surgical intervention. A typical complication among Crohn's patients.

Fissures – cuts (cracks) in the membrane that surrounds the anus. As a result of the tear the sphincter which closes the anus is exposed, something which causes spasm. The result is pain and bleeding during bowel movements.

Abscess – an accumulation of pus that is develops after infection and which can cause pain and temperature. A typical complication among Crohn's patients.

Malignant tumors – An active and continuous inflammation in the large intestine, increases the chances of bowel cancer.

External complications – The systems and tissues of organs outside of the digestive system such as joints, liver, skin, eyes and bones can suffer from inflammation or various complications as a result of the disease, or as a side effect of various drugs (mainly steroids). These external complications occur at lower rates of incidence.

Methods of treating the disease with medication

The aim of drug treatment is to suppress the inflammation and its symptoms and to prevent future recurrences. The doctor advises on the kind of drug treatment according to the severity of the inflammation and its location in the bowel. The treatment for Crohn's and Colitis are very similar.

Anti-inflammatories: Rafassal / Pentasa / Asacol / Salazopyrin / Dipentum. This group of drugs is known Aminosalycilates (5-ASA) [11] These work in a similar way to aspirin, with a local anti-inflammatory effect. They have been found to be efficient in treating Colitis, but opinion is divided about their efficiency in treating Crohn's disease. Because their side-effects are relatively light they are prescribed mainly to keep the inflammation in a state of inactivity – some in order to prevent attacks and a deterioration in the disease, and some to lessen the chance of a cancerous development in the large intestine that can occur during periods of active inflammation. The side-effects include, among other things, biliousness, dizziness, diarrhea, headache and joint pain.

Steroids: Budesonide / Prednisone [12] These are a kind "second track" in the treatment and are intended for a mid- to severe state of the disease. These steroids are hormones that are secreted naturally by the adrenal gland [13] (corticosteroids). They work to suppress the inflammatory process and their efficiency is proven.

---

[11] Aminosalicylic acid (5-ASA) www.medscape.com/viewarticle/556294

[12] www.drugs.com/prednisone.html www.drugs.com/mtm/budesonide.html

[13] The adrenal glands are located at the top of the kidneys and regulate the balance of many bodily functions by secreting hormones

Steroids have different strengths and the tendency is to use them minimally and for a short time. This is because of their severe side-effects which include, among other things, loss of calcium in the bones, diabetes, skin lesions, high blood pressure, increased weight, hirsutism, acne, disturbances in the immune system, sleep disorders, damage to the adrenal gland and so on. It is important to emphasize that side-effects vary among the different drugs. Despite the side-effects, there are cases when the use of steroids is definitely preferable to an active inflammation.

The relevant preparations are Prednisone and Budesonide which are taken as pills. It is possible to be treated with steroids by means of enemas – a method that reduces the side-effects (and which reaches the large intestine directly) – and in particularly severe cases, they can injected via a vein. Continued use of steroids is liable to develop a dangerous dependency. Steroids must be used in an enlightened way.

Drugs that suppress the immune system: Imuran / Purinethol / Methotrexate (6-MP) [14] These suppress the immune system, inhibit the disease and keep the inflammation in a state of remission [15]. They are even efficient in treating fistulae caused by the inflammation. In cases where the patient develops a dependency on steroids these drugs can help reduce or even stop their use. Apart from the field of bowel disease, these drugs are efficient in oncology treatments and also in treating patients who have undergone transplants. Their most noticeable disadvantage is the long time it takes for a response: From the moment when you begin taking the pill,

---

[14] Mercaptopurine, 6-MP, 6-Mercaptopurine (Purinethol), Azathioprine Imuran

www.drugs.com/cdi/azathioprine.html

www.drugs.com/cdi/mercaptopurine.html

[15] Remission is a state of calmness in which the symptoms of the disease disappear wholly or partially

it takes about three months before the effect is felt. More than that the suppression of bone marrow is expressed in a low white blood cell count – something that exposes the body to infection and requires high-frequency blood count and liver function monitoring in accordance with the doctor's instructions. The white blood cell count returns to normality after stopping the treatment. Apart from this the side-effects include, among other things, inflammation of the liver and pancreas and a lowering of fertility in men. It is recommended that pregnant women do not take these drugs, despite the fact that research has not proved that harm is caused to the fetus – with the exception of Methotraxate which is not allowed to be taken during pregnancy (it is recommended that you stop using the drug six months before conception. In Israel and Europe it is also recommended that men who take the drug do not impregnate their partners).

Anti-alpha TNF: Remicade / Humira / Cimzia [16]. These drugs include antibodies for cytokine alpha TNF, a substance that exists in the body and is active in processes that contribute to the outbreak of Crohn's disease. Taking this drug suppresses cytokine and inhibits the processes that cause the disease. Remicade works in a more focused and efficient way than Imuran because it in fact attacks the source of the inflammation. Remicade is prescribed once every two months as a transfusion into a vein and brings not only a remission but can even heal fistulae. However, its disadvantage is that the drug can increase the risk of lymphatic cancer and is liable to cause additional side-effects.

---

[16] Remicade / Humira/ Cimzia:

www.remicade.com/remicade/global/index.html

www.humira.com/CrohnsDisease/Default.aspx

www.cimzia.com/Default1.asp

Also, early exposure to tuberculosis is liable endanger the results of the treatment. Treatment with Remicaid is usually given alongside another treatment that suppresses immunity, such as 6-MP. A new drug by the name of Humira has now entered the market whose action resembles that of Remicaid but is given by a sub-cutaneous injection. Its advantage is that the patient does not have to go to hospital in order to get the injection. Cimnzia, whose action resembles that of Humira, is administered in the same way, with a sub-cutaneous injection.

Antibiotics: Ciproxin / Flagyl / Metrogel [17]
These are mostly anti-infection drugs that have been found to be efficient in treating bowel diseases. They are mostly given as a first option and short-term response to an acute inflammatory condition. The side-effects include neurological symptoms, biliousness and a metallic taste in the mouth. More extreme side-effects are the development of damage to the peripheral nervous system, and tingling in the soles of the feet. These drugs are given as a treatment for active inflammation of the small intestine, for fistulae and abscesses.

Important observations regarding treatment methods
As I have mentioned previously, the various treatments are not able to heal the disease. They can help the patient to achieve extended periods of calm and an improvement in the condition of the inflammation. The level of success depends on matching the treatment to the nature of the disease, which varies among patients. Often there is no real way of knowing if a particular treatment will succeed other than by trying it. It must be emphasized that although the drugs cannot heal the disease, suppression of the inflammation is

---

[17] Metronidazole:

www.drugs.com/metronidazole.html

no less important. The complications that are liable to cause damage that is much more serious than the side-effects of the drugs, and that result from an active inflammation, can be avoided by using the drugs.

In the past the treatment policy imposed order on the prescribing of drugs, from the lighter to the heavier: The patient began with Rafassal, moved on to steroids, and continued with Imuran and Remicade as the last resort. Today there is an approach that claims that the order should be reversed, and that one should rather begin with the stronger drugs to prevent the patient from reaching the stage of active inflammation and the extended use of steroids. I must mention that opinions in this regard are still divided.

Standard treatments for diarrhea are not recommended for patients with chronic diseases of the digestive system. These treatments have a direct effect on the working of the bowel. And they are not necessarily suited to the special needs of the patient.

Surgery

Surgery should be undertaken only in the case of complications: A lack of response to drug treatment, massive bleeding, treatment for serious fistulae and abscesses, dangerous and narrowing or blockage of the intestine. In situations like these, there is no alternative but to operate because of the lack of a medicinal treatment that could heal the condition with the required immediacy and effectiveness. As with drugs, an operation will never effect a full recovery, and is only a localized solution to a problem. The use of surgery as a means of prevention is therefore not recommended – the removal of the affected part of the bowel will not eradicate the disease, which in most cases will return to attack the bowel at the area of the surgery after about a year. Having said that, an operation which can prevent an emergency (such as a blockage of the intestine) and which can be done in controlled conditions, is preferable to an emergency operation for which there is less chance of success, and for which the recovery time is longer.

Diagnostic and monitoring systems

An updated picture of the state of the disease is a kind of jigsaw puzzle consisting of the patient's description and various tests, some of which I will detail here:

Blood test: A laboratory test of a blood sample from the patient's body. The test attempts to discover a number of relevant parameters of the disease such as the level of infection in the body, a lack of various dietary components, anemia (stemming from a lack of iron, B12, or folic acid), a cancerous development, problems with blood clotting, problems with bone marrow and so on. The test is relatively simple and is not accompanied by any particular danger.

Stool test: An additional laboratory test that does not endanger the patient. Its aim is to discover signs of infection especially in the large intestine involved in the disease. It is possible to discover signs of inflammation also in the small intestine by means of high levels of fat that testify to a lack of absorption.

Imaging tests:

X-ray – the use of x-rays to get an image of the hard tissue in the body. Imaging the digestive system is done by means of introducing a contrast medium (such as Barium), either by drinking it, or by means of a tube that goes from the nose to the stomach area, where the material is released to reach the bowel area to be x-rayed. The test confirms the diagnosis of Crohn's disease in the small intestine. With the x-ray it is possible to diagnose the state of the inflammation, to identify narrowing of the bowel and to locate fistulae and so on. Over-exposure to x-rays is not recommended, and they are not allowed for pregnant women.

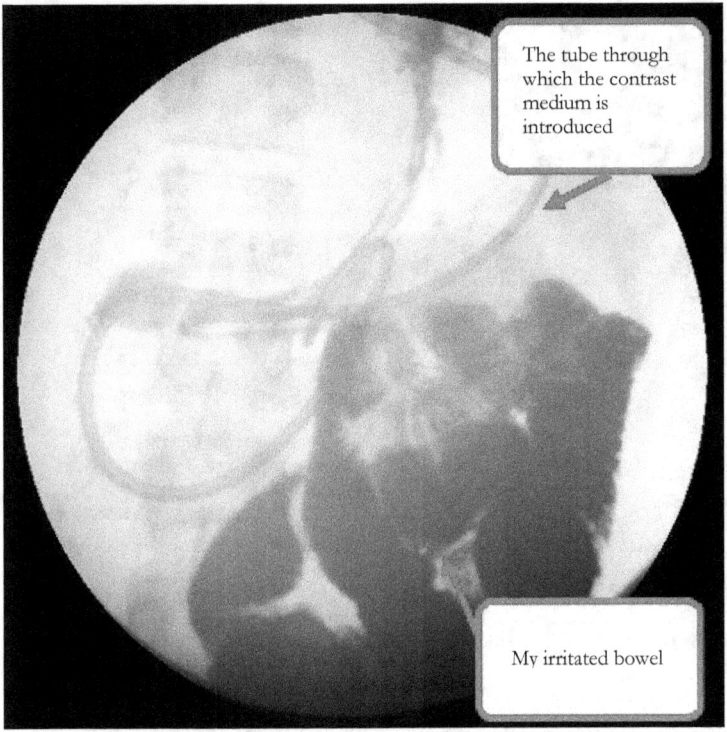

The tube through which the contrast medium is introduced

My irritated bowel

The X-ray image that I did as a part of my diagnosis during the period before my operation

- CT – Computerized tomography. A non-invasive image that is intended to provide a three-dimensional picture of the interior of the body. It is made by means of x-rays that are similar to normal x-rays and processed by computer to provide a three-dimensional picture of the body. This test allows for the identification of blocked areas of the bowel and liquids in the abdominal cavity. To do the test, it may be necessary to use a contrast medium which is introduced by drinking or by injection into a vein. Isolated exposure to the x-rays that are emitted during the test are not likely to cause any side-effects. However, multiple tests can have an impact on the seminal vesicles and in rare cases can even cause growths.

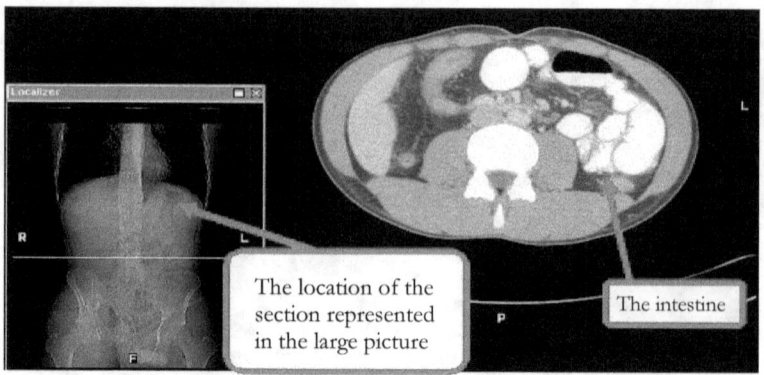

A cross-section of the bowel as revealed in the CT scan I did

- MRI – Magnetic resonance. A non-invasive scan that is used for imaging the interior of the body without the use of x-rays. This test is more exact than the CT scan and is accordingly more expensive. The test is based on radio waves that are reflected from the various tissues and which are processed in order to provide an image of the interior the body. The big advantage of the MRI scan, apart from its level of accuracy, is that it does not include radiation. The disadvantage is its high cost and the long queue of people waiting to do it.

Endoscopic tests: Endoscopy is a surgical procedure for a medical test on the human body by means of the introduction of a tube that contains an optical fiber and camera. The tube is introduced through the natural orifices of the body or via a cut in the skin (yes – just as it sounds, it hurts. You can request sedation). With this test it is possible to scan various internal organs: Esophagus, stomach and the digestive tract via the mouth (gastroscopy); the large intestine and the terminal part of the small intestine via the anus (colonoscopy); the bladder and urinary tract (cystoscopy), and so on. Tests of the organs connected to the digestive system are used mainly to diagnose various digestive diseases (among them Crohn's and Colitis), the discovery of ulcers and polyps and the removal of polyps. They therefore permit early discovery of cancerous growths and the identification of inflamed areas in the bowel. In general an endoscopy is used also for sampling tissues (biopsy) and internal operations.

The advantage of an endoscopy is the provision of a real-time picture of the area being checked (as opposed to imaging), and its ability to take a tissue sample from various areas (biopsy) – that can provide a more accurate diagnosis of the state of inflammation and cancerous cells. More than that, this test is considered to be safer because it doesn't include radiation that is damaging to the body.

*In most cases a Crohn's or Colitis patient needs to undergo the large intestine test by means of a colonoscopy. The most common routine includes drinking, on the day before the test, a liquid that causes diarrhea, being sedated before the tests begins (request as much as possible), and the insertion of a tube with the camera into the anus (yes – it's exactly what it sounds like).

According to Prof Fireman the danger of this test is that it can cause bleeding and perforation of the bowel, although the chances of this happening are very low, particularly if it's only a diagnostic test (without the excision of polyps). There are patients (myself among them) who believe that the test in fact causes a deterioration in the inflammation as a result of the irritation of sensitive areas. Having said that, you should not give up on the test, if only because of its ability to reveal the development of cancerous growths at an early stage. Patients with chronic diseases of the digestive system are among the group at risk of developing these growths. You will remember that Prof Fireman recommends doing this test once a year, beginning in the eighth year of the disease, and at any change in the disease. A small tip from my experience as a patient–it's desirable to reduce the amount you drink of the liquid that causes diarrhea, and rather fast for a little longer before the test. Aside from this, it's important, as far as it's possible, to make the correct choice of doctor to do the test. A test such as this one on an inflamed intestine which can so easily be injured, requires great skill and experience.

The pill camera: This is a relatively new test during which the patient swallows a miniature camera which photographs the digestive system for a number of hours, as it accompanies the food progressing from the mouth to the anus. From the point of view of the patient, this test is far simpler than an endoscopy and saves him all the discomfort. However, in this test it's not possible to take samples, and it's not recommended for patients suffering from an active infection because of the danger of a narrowing of the bowel or a blockage which may cause the camera to get stuck (something which would require surgery).

Recommended activities for Crohn's patients, beyond drug therapy

In cases where the disease spreads to more widespread areas and causes problems in the absorption of food in the body it is desirable for the patient to consume various vitamins in accordance with the deficiencies that have been determined by the blood test (absorption problems are not common when the disease is concentrated in the large intestine – an organ that is not responsible for absorption). It is desirable to supplement daily nutrition with a multi-vitamin that contains most of the vitamins required by the body. The levels of iron and vitamin B12 are particularly important, and a lack of them is typical of intestinal patients. Despite the unpleasantness, when there is an absorption problem, it's preferable to get the supplement via injection or infusion. It's necessary to take into account the fact that vitamin B12 tablets are liable to cause stomach pains in sensitive patients.

In cases of narrowing of the bowel, the narrowing does not permit the passage of some foods. The harder it is for food to be digested, the harder it will be for it to pass through the narrow area. This process is accompanied by pain and can even cause a blockage. In these situations the consumption of softer food (a low residue diet) is therefore recommended. You should keep fiber consumption to a minimum (avoid eating fresh fruit and vegetables) and increase liquid foods.

For small children or adolescents when there is a fear of developmental or growth impairment as a result of deficiencies (particularly common among users of steroids) – it is usual to recommend a low residue diet (a commercial dietary supplement designed to make up what the patient is lacking).

When the patient is admitted to hospital following an acute attack, it's usual to let the bowel rest with a diet introduced from outside of the body – that is, by means of infusion.

The way conventional medicine relates to alternative therapy

The intestinal patient suffers from a disease for which modern western medicine has no definite answers. The patient is required, over long periods, to gorge himself daily on pills. Gritting his teeth, he absorbs the side-effects, and is beyond frustration when it becomes clear that the pills don't help at all. The level of success of the treatment is unpredictable and to a degree, almost coincidental – certain patients will feel a change for the better, while others perhaps will not be affected. And if that were not enough, the conditions that accompany the treatment itself are far from satisfactory: The time devoted to each patient is short, the clinics are overloaded to the point of exhaustion, the lines are long, the treatments are repetitive, and the medication is not always effective. Given these circumstances, it's natural for the patient to feel that he is not getting a suitable response to his problems, and that the appropriate level of attention is simply not being invested in him. It's natural that he will explore other solutions for healing the disease.

Alternative treatment on the other hand, is characterized by the great amount of patience and attention that is granted to the patient. Beyond any assessment of the treatment itself, it's often through the psychological effect in the patient who feels that his problem is being treated with due seriousness, that he feels an improvement in his condition. This phenomenon is known as the placebo effect [18].

---

[18] Placebo effect: Improvement in the condition of a patient as a result of receiving a dummy drug or dummy treatment

It is important to point out that this psychological effect is subjective, and does not necessarily continue over an extended period, certainly for the diseases we are talking about. More than that, there have been cases where certain alternative treatments have even made the patient's condition worse, either because of the treatments themselves, or because of the change from conventional medical treatment. It is important to thoroughly check the capacity of the therapist and to ensure that you monitor your body's responses to the treatment. It goes without saying that any medical activity, including injections or surgery is better done by a qualified doctor.

What does the future hold?

Today tens of research programs are being conducted on bowel diseases, and their main aim is to find a drug for the disease. At the same time, the drugs that are available on the market are updated and improved periodically, so there is room for optimism.

Alternative medicine – Approaches to treatment and monitoring

With due respect to spirituality and lovers of nature, the most important thing is your health. Every treatment can help a healthy person. Every person will feel better if he gets attention, especially if he is paying for it. When you are really sick, you need to be more suspicious. You need to distinguish between a pleasant and interesting experience and an efficient treatment that also promotes health. Be honest with yourself – it doesn't matter how pleasant the therapist is, or how much he might have helped your sister-in-law to get rid of the rash on her back. If after a limited trial period during which you have tried all the aspects of the treatment, you don't feel an improvement, then just part as friends, and move on to another therapist, or different system of treatment. It's a waste of your time and money, and more than anything else – it's a waste in terms of your health.

The real importance of alternative treatments is, in my opinion, beyond the efficiency of the treatments themselves, the change from passivity to activity. The patient who has until this point plodded along with long waits in conventional treatment, and at the end of which he got the same old pill that doesn't necessarily help, is now suddenly taking responsibility for his health. The minute I decided "There is something that can be done!" I felt for the first time that I was doing something to heal myself. The decision to stop waiting for the drugs to do the work was an important landmark in my struggle to deal with the disease.

The hope and belief that flowed from this change could by themselves have brought about the hoped-for improvement and the success of the treatment.

About crooks and thieves

I'll tell you a secret. Not every person who seems spiritual or connected with nature, and who manages a beautiful and well-ordered clinic flooded with the pleasant scent of incense and posters of the human body divided into slices and meridians, knows what he is doing. The alternative medicine market is full of crooks and I'm sure that the professionals in the field will agree with me on this. If by any chance you have come across one of these crooks, the loss of your money is liable to be the least of your woes. Just as there are treatments that can help, there are those that can cause damage. Therefore, even before you start the treatment it's important to clarify some important details about the therapist (either via recommendations or direct questions): Where did he study? How long has he been practicing? Does he have experience in the field in which your problem is to be found? Most important of all is to know that you can always leave a treatment in the middle. Remember that if a treatment fails, it doesn't necessarily mean a failure of the field itself – it's entirely possible that the failure is due only to the low level of expertise of the therapist.

The special characteristics of Crohn's and Colitis that include the absence of effective drugs, symptoms whose sources and strength are difficult to describe accurately, and the connection between the severity of the disease and one's mental state – all these are fertile ground for alternative treatments. The therapist can easily gain the patient's trust – sometimes without real foundation. Like many other patients, I am prepared to try just about any treatment that might help me to overcome the disease. It was within the framework of these experiments that over the years I passed through the hands of tens of alternative practitioners across a considerable number of more or less well-known fields of treatment. The only clear conclusion that has come out of all these years is that there is no healing drug for Crohn's disease. There are many kinds of treatments that can help the disease subside for a certain time and even achieve a remission of years, but anyone who promises that he has the power to heal you of the disease – flee from him as you would from fire!

I don't mean to discourage you with this pile of warnings. I have no doubt that a patient who is interested in improving his condition has to incorporate alternative treatment alongside the conventional. It requires care and patience but it will definitely pay off.

The issues I'll be presenting in the following chapters come from my personal experience as a patient. Some of them improved my condition, and some had no effect at all or even made things worse. In any event this information doesn't provide a comprehensive and professional picture of the huge variety of alternative treatments that are out there – it's intended as a recommendation only. I really hope that it will help you find the treatment system and the therapist that suit you.

A specialist in food supplements

Food supplements are there to complement the essential components that the body does not manage to produce from the food we consume: Vitamin B12, folic acid, iron, and so on. Food supplements come as pills, powder and various liquids. Treatment in this field requires consuming a great number of them to help the body deal with the disease.

Most Crohn's patients whose disease manifests in the small intestine suffer from absorption problems. Correct nutrition alone is therefore not enough to supply the body with everything it needs, and it's necessary to balance what is lacking with supplements. There are however disadvantages with this field of treatment. Firstly, too much, rather than gradual, consumption of supplements may place a burden on the body and disturb the already delicate balance in the system.

The inflammation, as you know, does not respond well to change, something that is likely to lead to a deterioration of the disease. Secondly the cost is far from negligible, particularly when you're talking about the large quantities that the body requires for supplementation. And finally, the difficulty with such intensive consumption of pills (alongside the conventional treatment) causes many to abandon the treatment after only a few weeks.

My recommendation:

In my experience, and that of other Crohn's patients, it's better not to load the digestive system with large amounts of supplements, and thus preserve time, money and health. Sometimes not all the supplements available on the market are suited to Crohn's patients. There are even some which can cause deterioration of the inflammation and pain. You should carefully select a quality preparation, and try it out gradually and in a controlled way. If after a trial period you feel no improvement, it's desirable that you stop. Having said that, you should not give up complementing the substances you need. After you do periodic blood tests, in consultation with a doctor you can decide on which supplements it's worth focusing. It's generally preferable to concentrate on single preparations such as multi-vitamins over a long period. Other important supplements are iron, vitamin B12, folic acid, and pro-biotic bacteria. You can find all these supplements at any pharmacy.

Some tips

Iron – It is desirable to take Gentle Iron, because normal iron under certain circumstances is likely to cause pain. Vitamin B12 – You can take it in the form of pills for dissolving under the tongue in order to enable absorption via the oral cavity instead of the damaged intestine. There are also oral sprays, but they cost more. If these substances are lacking in your body in especially high quantities, you can get them via injection or infusion.

Guided imagery

In the process of guided imagery, the therapist guides the patient on how to use his imagination to arrive at a personal consciousness and interiority. With this it's possible to isolate problematic elements that lead ultimately also to physical problems. The treatment process usually begins with light meditation with the emphasis on breathing. In the subsequent treatments the patient is guided on how to activate various images that allow him to sense and control different physical feelings. Within this framework, the technique of returning the patient to various situations from the course of his life may be used.

My recommendation:

As I have already mentioned, after many years of struggling with a chronic active inflammation, I am convinced of the direct connection between the severity of the inflammation and one's mental state. During all the periods of my life when I was stressed I always felt less well than during periods when I was calmer and more at peace. The equation, as I have said, works both ways. In order to improve one's physical condition, it's desirable to treat it by means of the mind. Alternative treatments in general, and guided imagery in particular, emphasize treating the mind. It's not at all certain that this method will suit everyone, but with the help of the right therapist and a positive and open approach, it's possible to produce good tools for calming and healing.

Homeopathy

This is one of the most popular treatment methods. According to the homeopathic approach, a person is a whole entity in which there exists a tight connection between body and mind. Hence the treatment does not focus on specific symptoms of the disease, but rather on one's general state of health and mind. The treatment includes giving natural remedies that have no chemical ingredients. Made by means of a repeated and changing dilution of their constituents, they are individually matched to the patient by the homeopath and with their energy, awaken the patient's own natural healing power.

My recommendation:
Despite homeopathy's popularity I do not have positive personal experience of the treatment. I can't point to any homeopathic therapist or remedy that improved my condition. However, because we're speaking here about natural substances only, there is no real danger of deterioration. It's therefore definitely worth at least trying.

Camel milk

Camel milk probably contains substances that assist the functioning of the immune system, as well as various fats that contribute to the development of the brain and the nerves. Moreover, it is claimed that camel's milk has the ability to heal inflammatory diseases, among them, Crohn's and Colitis. You can order the milk frozen in plastic bottles directly to your house – you then thaw it and drink it twice a day in varying amounts.

My recommendation:
Various sources have claimed to me that camel milk helps Crohn's patients to suppress the inflammation. It could be that this comes from the fact that these patients consume the milk in place of cow's milk, which is known for making the disease worse. I tried camel milk for quite a while, but regretfully never found the wonder drug. Because so many recommend it, and because its taste is not bad at all (certainly in comparison with other potions I have tasted), and its price is not particularly high – it's worth trying. Perhaps its magic will work for you.

Chinese medicine

This is the most ancient therapeutic system in the field of alternative medicine, and developed from Chinese culture and philosophy about four thousand years ago. In a very general sense Chinese philosophy looks at the person as an integral part of the world in which he lives, and the person must therefore live in harmony with that world and the changes that continually take place in it (changes of season, temperature, and so on). The treatment systems attempt to "balance" the patient with the nature around him. The various treatments include acupuncture [19], treatment with healing herbs, touch therapy (Tui Na, Shiatsu) and others.

Acupuncture is the most common treatment. It balances bodily energy by means of introducing extremely narrow needles at acupuncture points that are found on channels (meridians) along which the energy (ch'i) flows. To find out more about Chinese medicine and its connection with Crohn's disease, please see the chapter Alternative Medicine – Chinese Medicine and Crohn's disease.

My recommendation:
I wholeheartedly recommend it! I have no idea how it works. I don't know which ch'i flows where. However, after a few failed therapists (among them even some real Chinese ones) I found the one who worked for one hour a week in releasing me from pain and stopping the diarrhea. Altogether I feel better after every treatment, and for a patient who suffers permanently from pain that is really not a small thing. You don't have to experience the entire history of Chinese treatments – you make do just with acupuncture or Tui Na (even without herbs).

---

[19] Acupuncture - From the Latin "needle", the "points" at which needles are inserted

What is most important is that you choose a serious therapist who gives you the full attention you need. As long as I'm recommending things – for patients who suffer from pains in various areas it's worth trying Moxa [20]. This is a cigar-shaped roll, not at all expensive, which is used to heat a painful area – and believe me, it works wonders.

Reflexology

Reflexology makes use of the feet to diagnose and treat various diseases. The treatment includes pressure, movement and heating of various areas of the foot that radiate out to different areas of the body. According to this teaching, every organ of the body corresponds to an area on the foot. And the connection runs in both directions. When a particular area is injured or if its energy is blocked (the blockages are known as crystals), it is felt as a hardening of the corresponding area on the foot.

My recommendation:
On the one hand, this system can certainly help to conquer the pain. On the other hand, when you become a little more familiar with it, it's definitely possible to harness a trustworthy family member to the task, and thereby save on the cost of a professional therapist. It lends itself to self-study from books and of course by trial and error. With a little experience it's possible to feel where the painful areas are located and to free them with the help of the correct pressure. There is a lot of information on the internet for those who want to gain expertise in the field.

---

[20] Moxa (from Chinese medicine): A cigar-shaped roll that contains a mixture of herbs for burning, and that enables heating and calming in painful areas.

Western herbal medicine

Western herbal medicine is similar to Chinese medicine in its use of the healing power of herbs but with the emphasis on those plants that grow in western countries. Some of the plants have the ability to heal diseases and various sores (the Aloe Vera plant, for example, has the ability to heal sores and irritations on the skin). Various solutions or powders that are easy to consume are prepared from the relevant plants.

My recommendation:

There is no doubt that plants have features that can affect our bodies and health. The various drugs that are produced from plants and the fact that it's forbidden to grow them are a more than good indication of this. Alongside these plants, there are many that can ease inflammation and infection, strengthen the body and calm the spirit. It's desirable that you get to know and use the basic plants that help in calming the digestive system, for example, like the herb chamomile. A dried chamomile infusion improves the digestive process and can help in calming inflammation. You can find a lot of information on the plants on the internet and in various books, but in this case I recommend consulting with a qualified therapist who can help and direct the treatment in ways that suit you.

Naturopathy

Naturopathy includes a number of fields, among them healing herbs, nutrition, homeopathy and more. In this area, the patient's nutrition is matched to his blood type. There are four blood types: A, B, AB or O. According to the principles of naturopathy each one of these groups is suited to different diets such as useful foods that one should increase, neutral foods that one should eat in moderation, and harmful foods that one should not eat at all. With the aid of correct nutrition – which as I have mentioned is one of the most important elements in coping with the disease –you can strengthen the immune system, improve the metabolism, prevent infections and improve your health.

My recommendation:
After a personal experience of failure that included a deterioration in health and the loss of not a little money, I can't recommend the method. I believe that there is no therapist who can say to a Crohn's patient exactly what the optimum diet for him should be. Only the patient, on his own, on the strength of his own experience, can decide that. For certain patients the disease and the bowel behave in a different way, and they therefore respond differently to certain foods – this despite the fact that they have the same blood type. Accordingly, their diet needs to be different. For those patients who would nevertheless like to try it, I would recommend that before beginning the treatment you check your blood type yourself with a simple blood test, and make use of the streams of information that flow across the internet and the literature on this subject (you can put together detailed nutritional tables on your own according to this method). In my view, you should save valuable money and time.

Garlic concentrate

The capacity of garlic for healing has been known in various cultures from the dawn of history. It is even known as "nature's antibiotic" and it is claimed that it has the power to heal infections and inflammations, and even to strengthen the immune system. There are foods that contain concentrated essences of garlic. Taking a few drops a day provides the body with this healing power, and it does indeed have a significant effect.

My recommendation:
I believe in the capacity of various plants to affect our bodies, certainly to no less a degree than chemicals. In the right doses garlic can help in the struggle with the disease as it is defined as an

111

inflammation that is accompanied by various infections along the length of the digestive system. Having said this, I don't think you should rush out and buy special products so that you can enjoy garlic's therapeutic capacity. It's enough to incorporate completely normal, fresh garlic as a permanent ingredient of your daily menu. There are those who claim that only fresh garlic contains the necessary active ingredients and that you should consume a clove of fresh garlic a day. Another possibility is to crush a clove of garlic, leave it to soak in water for some time, and then drink it. I admit and confess that I have tried, and ceased, this custom – something to do with the combination of the horrible taste and the strange need that people have to keep to a distance greater than five meters away from me.

Magnets

During my search for medication I came across a system of therapy which uses magnets. There is a claim according to which a magnetic field helps in some way in the healing of various diseases, and among them, Crohn's.

My recommendation:
Lo and behold, hocus pocus! My money was attracted to the therapist's wallet! It seems as if the system works. At least it didn't damage my health.

Lasers

Lasers are used for various medical needs such as eliminating the need for spectacles, and in various plastic surgery applications. In the last few years a branch of treatment has developed which makes use of lasers also for treating external pain and infection. Although this mostly deals with pain that stems from orthopedic problems, nevertheless, after my operation I decided to try this treatment to overcome the pain of Crohn's. The treatment consisted of the radiation of a number of laser beams of varying wavelength and frequency over the injured area.

My recommendation:

After my operation I suffered from infection in the area of the main cut. This infection did heal – possibly as a result of using the laser, but it was also possibly due to the anti-infection ointments that I used. However, with everything that has to do with internal pain and inflammation, the laser treatment did not help, and might just possibly have made the situation worse. I would not recommend trying treatment of this type until proven experience has been accumulated in the field.

Countless solutions and potions

Every therapist who respects himself will always try to sell you the "wonder drug" that will heal the disease at precisely the same speed that he swipes your credit card. What these drugs have in common, whether they are made up from plants or prepared from other substances, is their awful taste and a texture that makes them difficult to swallow. Even if you find the magician (the therapist) who will succeed in giving you a drug whose taste and texture is as wonderful as French vanilla ice cream, don't ever give up on the truly important test – which active ingredients does it contain and whether they can improve or strengthen your health.

My recommendation:

Don't ever be a guinea-pig for therapists who have no experience of your disease, or for therapists who have experience and try out new methods of treatment on desperate patients. Don't give up on important checks regarding your therapist and his background, and don't accept every "drug" for going through your digestive system. Even if you've paid for an expensive and quality product, don't hesitate to throw it in the trash can if your condition deteriorates after a while. The money you will lose is not worth the price you will pay with your health.

The rule of thumb in choosing a treatment method and therapist

Any drug that worsens the situation already at the beginning will never contribute to an improvement in the future (even if the therapist tells you otherwise). Having said that – in cases where there is no deterioration you need to be patient and give it time, even if there is no real improvement at the beginning. There are treatments whose effects require time to evaluate.

Stay away from anyone who claims that he has a wonder drug or treatment that will cause the disease to disappear. There are of course various drugs and treatments that provide long periods of a relaxation of the disease so that it will seem as if it has disappeared exactly as it came. Often it is turns out be an illusion that can deaden your caution mechanisms and disrupt your habits. The attack, which won't be late in coming, will very quickly bring you back to reality.

If it feels expensive, it probably is expensive. In my experience the best therapists are not necessarily the most expensive. Mostly, as you might expect, a therapist who sets a high price on his expertise will not devote himself entirely to the patient.

If a therapist tells you to take more than three medications, either pills or solutions, that is exactly the time to start asking questions. I have come across not a few therapists who market their own drugs or who are connected to one or another pharmacy, who try to grab profits on your account. When you weigh up the cost of the treatment, you should also take the medication into account.

You should stay away from any therapist who interferes with the conventional medical treatment – every therapist should concentrate on the field he knows.

You need to try every new treatment gradually so that you can check its effect on your body.

Do not try any pill, solution or drink that doesn't have a "mother or father" – there is no need to experiment with every medication or plant that someone has found on a picnic near some town in the boondocks – and certainly not those that do not have a responsible therapist or organized treatment system behind them. Remember it's easy to do great damage.

Listen to your body before you listen to any therapist.

"Life is pain. Anyone who says differently is selling something"
William Goldman, *The Princess Bride.*

In sum

One of the serious effects of the proliferation of charlatans in the field of alternative medicine is the phenomenon of the rejection by many patients of this treatment who despair after a number of unsuccessful attempts. These patients completely abandon alternative medicine and place their confidence only in conventional medicine. Remember that the path to finding the therapeutic method and the therapist that suit you is one of continuous pain and disappointment. It is enough, however, that one therapist succeed in finding the right method in order to work wonders with the state of your disease and your feelings. Don't give up – do everything to learn, read on the internet, and accept recommendations from patients. The effort will pay off. Your body is worth the quest.

"The Prince should ask his advisers about everything and listen to their opinions – and afterwards decide on his own in his own way ..." Niccolo Machiavelli, *The Prince* [i]

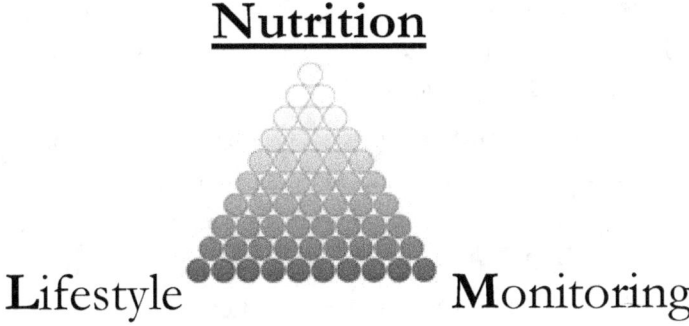

Nutrition (LM**N**)

You are what you eat!

When I was fifteen years old and I was diagnosed with Crohn's disease they explained to me that it was an inflammation of the bowel which is part of the digestive system, and that as a result of this I would have to adapt myself to various eating habits. "No problem", I said, "just tell me what's permitted and what's not, and I'll keep to a correct diet and everything will be alright."

After a conversation with the doctor who diagnosed me with the disease, a medical insurance dietician and a range of clerks and other officials at the health institutions, I managed to make the following summarized list of problematic foods:

- Spicy is forbidden – "because it burns you bowel".
- Everything that includes fiber is forbidden – "because it scratches the bowel wall". That meant vegetables and fruit were not allowed (especially citrus fruits) as well as whole-wheat bread and other foods that contain fibers. Tomatoes, eggplants and peppers were forbidden

also, as foods that contain fiber, and more than that, because "they are too acidic". Naturally ketchup was out of the question, and if you thought about it – the same went for all other herb products as well.

- Meat is not recommended because "it is hard to digest".
- White sugar – "not recommended because it encourages inflammation, and is anyway generally not healthy". It's true of all foods of course, that they contain sugar, especially all the sweetened drinks. White bread was also not recommended because of the white flour it contains.
- Everything that contains preservatives is forbidden – because "with them the food remains in the intestine and can encourage inflammation".
- Everything that contains food coloring is forbidden – "because it is simply not healthy".
- Every fizzy drink is forbidden – "because as it stands we already have enough gas in the bowel". Cola, from which it was very hard for me to part, of course contains both sugar and food coloring. The prohibitions on fiber and sugar left me with a glassful of water.
- It's not recommended to eat out – "because it's not clean".
- Fried foods – "not healthy".
- Dairy products – "not recommended because they are not digested well and can encourage diarrhea".
- Pulses such as chick-peas and broad beans – they cause gas and are therefore not worth it.

After all the conversations, consultations and the lists, I was left, as you can see, with rice and water. The doctors of course added that it was important to eat a lot because I was very thin and needed lots of vitamins so that my body could cope with the disease.

After a week of a strict and depressing diet, I celebrated its sooner than expected end at McDonalds.

Setting aside the cynicism, I admit that the advice that I got was not wrong. It is all correct in principle, but of course one needs to follow it in moderation. First and foremost, you need to understand that Crohn's is not a disease for lazy people (in the end it will turn out that excess diligence will be the real reason for the disease...). Also and mainly, from a nutritional point of view, there is no alternative to hard work. Every patient has to make an investment and learn by himself which types of food are good for him, and which are not. After long years of treatment, and ups and downs, it seems that the best advice I got from any doctor ever was "eat everything you want, and if something gives you a sore stomach, don't eat it again." In the end, you are for yourself and your health, and as the wise man used to say: "Listen to everyone's advice, but take your own decisions."

The great problem with the subject of nutrition stems from the gap between what is forbidden and the many constraints, and the body's need for essential nutritional elements (vitamins, minerals and so on). What is even more serious for patients is that their disease is active in the small intestine, something that causes absorption problems. Thus, even if your nutrition is appropriate, balanced and contains all the required nutritional components, you will still encounter deficiencies. Many Crohn's patients therefore suffer from a deficiency of iron, vitamin B12, folic acid, zinc and calcium. Similarly, not a few suffer from malnutrition and weight-loss. This gap obliges every patient whose health is important to him to thoroughly know the state of his health so that he can consume most of the nutrients his body needs while making the least possible mistakes.

Despite the fact that every patient responds differently to various types of foods, it's possible to define a number of common guidelines for correct nutrition:

No eating out

Long before the question "What should I eat?" comes the question "Where should I eat?" I'll try to be as clear as possible on this matter because people sometimes have a tendency to distort things. Repeat aloud after me, and practice with me the most important rule of nutrition: "I will never be tempted to eat out!" Repeat this mantra three times a day – there's a chance that you'll start to feel better. I know at first-hand that this is a harsh sentence, and not just from the point of view of entertainment and indulgence. It's also from a practical point of view that it seems impossible. Most people are not at home for most of the hours in a day, and they can't return home every time they want to snack on something. I'm definitely aware of the problematic nature of this. I live it. However, as I indicated earlier – this is not a disease for lazy people, and the solutions require investment.

Eating out endangers your health for the simple reason that you can never control the quality of every ingredient that appears before you on the plate. An unsuccessful dish that would cause an ordinary member of the community no more than a little gas, could send us to the emergency room within half an hour. I must emphasize that it makes no difference how clean the place is, and how nice the people there are. It could be any restaurant, any cafeteria, any fast food stand or any kiosk that sells popcorn for the movies. It can happen even if the owner cleans the kitchen three times a day (something he doesn't do), and even if he verifies that the person making the snack remembered to wash his hands after going to the bathroom (and who knows if he did so). It's enough that one single tiny pickled cucumber has had enough of its miserable life in the jar. Such a cucumber, already not fresh, becomes a large dwelling for germs. All on its own, as part of the wonderful and sterile "health helping" that you ordered, it can get you into deep trouble. Our angry bowels are just looking for a reason to get irritated, and the quality of the food is an excellent reason. Even if you don't feel the results immediately, an angry bowel has the memory of an elephant. It will not forget, and will definitely not forgive, the unnecessary bite you gave to a dying cucumber.

You will say, and rightly so, that home food is also not sterile. Having said that, because we know exactly what the level of sterility is and what the best ingredients are (and we can ensure a high level that suits our needs) we can minimize the danger significantly. Likewise, when the person preparing the food does it in the knowledge that the customer is the owner of a sensitive digestive system, it's clear that the ingredients and the herbs will be suitable.

And when you do go out? It's very simple: we take food and drink with us – sandwiches that will keep you going at your studies until the afternoon, or a container of food to heat up in the microwave at work. True – it's not always the tastiest, and it's definitely less simple and pleasant. "Not for lazy people," did I say? I promise that you'll thank yourselves in the evenings, when your stomach remains calm.

The ban, my friends, is in place when you're enjoying yourself at a restaurant. Do your best to make do with a light dish and a drink. Remember that even if someone else is paying the bill, you will pay the price for every mistake – with your health. For those of you who can't help yourselves, or when there is simply no alternative, do yourselves a favor: reduce the amount, and avoid experimenting with new dishes and with adventures at the expense of your intestines. Even in cases where you have to eat out, keep fast foods out of the picture, and choose from among the better quality restaurants.

Learn to cook

Just as a diabetes patient learns to use syringes and needles to inject himself with insulin; just as a celiac patient learns to look for the gluten in every food he consumes – in the same way Crohn's and Colitis patients need to become proficient in everything connected with food, and yes – learn to cook. We have to know exactly what's in every single thing that we put into our mouths, and to adapt ourselves to habits of checking the ingredients and expiration date of every product. It is only in this way that we'll be able to discover which ingredients are problematic for us, and it's only in this way that we'll know to guard against them in the future.

Despite the negative viewpoint, you must never forget that food is one of the greatest joys of life. You have to discover what you can eat, and to vary your menu as much as possible. If the menu is not varied and tasty enough, you will lose your appetite and you won't eat enough, and worse than that, you will be tempted to find easy and harmful solutions.

As I mentioned in the chapter in which I discussed lifestyle, cooking can also benefit you psychologically – both as occupational therapy and out of a sense that you are taking responsibility for your health – being proactive for the sake of your health as opposed to the passivity of taking medication and following the instructions of the doctors blindly.

Small meals with high frequency

The digestive system of bowel patients is very sensitive, and therefore should not be overburdened, even if it's with healthy, quality food. Give the system small amounts that it can deal with. Eat a little, but with high frequency. Eating large meals is an unhealthy custom for any person, and most certainly for bowel patients. In addition, it's desirable to stop eating a moment before the stomach is completely full – when the feeling of satiety is just beginning to appear.

Nutritional Agenda

It's important to ensure daily nutritional planning. When you go out of the house for an extended period, it's important to take sandwiches or food in a container to avoid as far as possible arriving at a state of hunger. That kind of situation is dangerous for a number of reasons. (1) When you are hungry, your judgment concerning what you should eat becomes blurred. A situation like this increases the chances of giving in to the temptation of food not prepared at home, or food of lesser quality. (2) Most bowel patients are not overweight, which means that their reserves are relatively diluted. Hunger is just one step before bodily collapse. (3) Hunger tends to lead to a large meal the next time you do eat. And large meals are not recommended for owners of a sensitive bowel.

The daily struggle over the amount of food that we consume is extremely important. There is a tendency to eat less when there is pain and diarrhea, something that can cause fatigue in our bodies. In accordance with what I said in the last paragraph, I recommend that you spread the amount of food you eat over the whole day, and not concentrate it, especially not towards the end of the day. I recommend that you reduce your eating before sleep, and in this way allow your system to rest and the body to enjoy a calm sleep without pain and stress. Eat only food prepared at home, but if you have to eat out it's important to know exactly where it will be so that you can avoid disastrous spontaneity. Yes, it's boring, but the disease loves routine, and we love life.

We pay for every mistake

You cannot play with nutrition. You will pay with your health for every wrong decision, even if it's in ways that are not immediately apparent. The accumulated damage that is caused to the system as a result of poor nutrition will also cause you to regret every time that you gave up when it came to food. Be honest with yourself – know which food is not good for you and don't eat it again. There is no dish in the world that is worth the deterioration of your health.

Let the system rest

The digestive system (yours in particular) needs rest, especially in light of the fact that it is active for most of the day. Do your best to calm the system a good few hours before you go to sleep. About three hours before going to bed it's desirable to consume mainly liquids and food that is easy to digest and to prepare the system for complete rest during sleep. Just as you need rest in front of the television or with a good book at the end of a hard day, so should you also give your digestive system a chance to recover from the hardships of the day.

Try on your own

The directive regarding spicy food, preserved food, or low-quality food is simple – it's out of the question. The decision concerning most other types of food is not so clear-cut. All might go smoothly with a particular food for a particular patient, yet wreak havoc in the stomach of another. The reason is the complexity of the intestine and the location of the inflammation which differs from patient to patient, with time, and even within the bowel of each patient himself. Every patient therefore must learn which foods are good for him and which are likely to make the state of the disease worse.

The only way to do this is via trial and error, but try to ensure that the 'error" part will be as small as possible. Introduce an item of any given food gradually and in an isolated manner into your menu, and check the response of your system in the hours following the meal. It's important to take note of every sound and feeling in your stomach, not to mention of course any diarrhea and pain. In my experience the real problem of this check is actually psychological. It's very difficult for people to admit that a particular food that they love is not good for them. However, we need to remember that the obligation to discover and research lies with you, and in order to succeed you have to be honest. It is only through honesty and awareness of the fact that you have to take that wonderful dish that you love off your menu, that you will succeed in avoiding a colossal catastrophe in the toilet after each meal. It is important not to give up on adding new items to your menu, otherwise it will be difficult to maintain nutritional discipline.

It's not just the disease, but the studies too that are dynamic. It's very possible that your correct diet will change over the years. With time and experience you will become your own best dieticians, and you will know by yourself which foods are good for you and which you should not eat, and you will even be able to quickly adapt to changes.

The senses as sensors

Our bodies contain many senses and we need to learn how to use them. When it comes to food, this is extremely important, especially for those of us who are the owners of sensitive digestive systems.

Smell – You need to use your sense of smell without any sense of shame or guilt. Smell the dishes that are presented to you, from milk to fish. Using it is important for example in identifying the early stages of decay in meat, chicken and fish. Even if it only smells a little bad, don't eat it, and it doesn't matter how prestigious it is. There is only one reason why the food smells bad, and it's not such a good one. Your stomach will also be quite resolute on this issue, believe me.

Taste – You can immediately feel on the tongue whether a dish is too spicy, too sour or too hot. The burning sensation in the oral cavity is a warning sign to us that the food that we are about to swallow in another few seconds is not good for our bodies.

Sight – A dish that doesn't look good testifies to its quality. It's especially true when you eat out. Pay attention to the general state of hygiene in the place (which is usually a reflection of the state of the kitchen), as well as to the look of the dish that you are getting, of course. Just about every food product can reveal its condition by its look – freshness, rottenness, level of sterility and so on. Open your eyes and in time your senses will get sharper.

Start your day gently

After you get up in the morning it's desirable to also allow your digestive system to wake up calmly. Begin the day with a hot drink, preferably tea or an infusion, and move to something light like a slice of bread or toast. After a few minutes you can continue with heavier things (but still with care!).

Hot is preferable to cold

On the recommendation of a number of alternative therapists, I adopted the rule according to which hot food and drink is preferable to cold. The digestive system responds better to these kinds of dishes, especially in cases of inflammation and narrowing of the bowel. It's possible that this is connected with the fact that heat expands the blood vessels, and cold shrinks them. I must emphasize that I'm not saying that you should take cold foods off your menu, only that you should reduce the amount you consume, especially in cases of active inflammation.

Know the ingredients of every product

Create a habit for yourself: read the label on every product that you buy, and check what it's made up of. You should avoid substances that are not natural like food coloring and preservatives. Remember that when there is doubt there is no doubt: if you come across strange names of ingredients that you don't know, you can safely assume that they are not natural ingredients, and therefore also not particularly healthy. The order in which the ingredients appear on the label is also very important. The ingredient that appears first is the one of which the product contains the greatest amount; the second is found in a lesser quantity and so on.

Preservatives

There are substances that are known not to be particularly healthy, and even less so for patients suffering digestive system problems. Preservatives are among the most prominent of these substances, and as their name implies, they preserve the food so that it won't decay and rot. The problem is that the preserving does not end at the moment of swallowing, but continues also inside the body causing the food not to be digested properly. The result is an increase in food residues in the digestive system. It is therefore recommended to avoid, as far as possible, products that contain preservatives (pastrami, sausage and yellow cheese, among others).

Beef

This is a sensitive subject for every lover of beef who suffers from a disease of the digestive system. In meat there are many essential substances such as iron, protein, B12, and fats that are lacking in the bodies of many Crohn's patients. But before these substances there is an even more difficult problem – meat is simply tasty, and someone who is used to consuming it on a daily basis will find it hard to part from it. The problem for Crohn's patients is that meat is hard to digest, and its passage through the digestive system requires a lot of time and resources. Moreover, meat, as it is sold today in all its different forms is very likely to contain organisms that cause a deterioration in the inflammation. Therefore, and with a heavy heart, I have to admit that meat is indeed a problematic item on the menu, and it is desirable to reduce its consumption to a minimum. If you can't resist it, at least insist on quality and on small amounts, in particular to make it easy on the system.

Chicken

People need to eat, and for someone who has to give up meat on the menu, chicken is not a bad substitute. Chicken can provide the energy that is lacking for us as patients, while at the same time being easier to digest than beef. More than that, chicken can be very tasty – even more so than meat – if you put some effort into it. However, before you pounce on the nearest chicken run, it's advisable even with chicken, not to overdo it. It's preferable to eat fish, but for those who insist it's better to make do with three portions a week, in small amounts (free-range chicken is preferable, not fried and without side dishes).

Fish

After we have finished with the negative side of the ten commandments of diet, we can happily move to the positive side – what is allowed, and even worth eating: fish should be the main item on your menu. We're talking about every kind of fish (sea-fish are preferable), as long as they are fresh and perfectly cooked. Fish is easy to digest and rich in proteins essential for the body. For the sake of comparison, the digestion time for fish is on average twice as fast as for chicken, and five times as fast as for meat. While these figures are true for a healthy person, the relative ratios remain more or less the same also for ourselves, the patients. More than that, fish dishes are rich in fish oil that contains omega 3 (yes, exactly the same supplement from the advertisements, only better because it comes in its natural form). The omega 3 acids have a hugely positive effect on the immune system in preventing inflammation in the body and even cancerous growths. Similarly these acids are responsible for the production of many balancing substances and processes in our bodies – blood pressure, temperature, inflammations, welling, pain and so on. Thus, for Crohn's patients, there are great benefits in consuming fish, both dietary and medical.

Eggs

I have yet to meet a patient who claimed that eating eggs caused him digestive problems. As opposed to other protein-rich foods such as chicken or meat, eggs are usually digested properly and supplement the missing energy that results from the eating of less chicken and meat. Even when I have had an acute attack with pain, when every other food only encouraged the inflammation, the eating of soft-boiled eggs never caused problems for me. The opposite is true – eggs helped return energy to the body, and even produced a feeling of fullness. Eggs cooked in different forms are recommended for your weekly menu.

Milk

For various reasons many people are sensitive to products produced from cow's milk. Officially, Crohn's and Colitis patients are not described as among these, but in my experience milk is difficult to digest, and even promotes diarrhea. In Dr Arieh Avni's book Fools of Milk [vii] he describes how an organism that is found in cow's milk causes many diseases, among them Crohn's. *"I have determined that Crohn's disease is caused by the infection in people by the organism MAP, that is found in cow's milk and its products."*

Also: *"Today with sophisticated methods the organism can be identified in between fifty to eighty percent of all patients... milk is contaminated by what generates the disease. If you do not touch milk products – you will not see Crohn's disease..."*

It must be pointed out that no proven connection has been found in research between Crohn's disease and the consumption of dairy products. It is important to know that there is a high frequency of a lack of lactose [21] among Crohn's patients, and therefore, in cases where milk is avoided, it is necessary to supplement the diet with vitamin D and calcium.

I recommend approaching cow's milk and its products with suspicion and trying them with caution. Milk is also forbidden in the Specific Carbohydrate Diet (see below). For those who are sensitive there are substitutes in the form of goat's milk and soya milk (see also camel milk in the sub-section that deals with alternative medicine). Today there is a wide range of products that make a good substitute for cow's milk in cheeses, delicatessen products, and milk in cartons. It's easy to find them on the shelves, and after you try them, you'll find that most are even more tasty.

Rice

Rice is healthy and nutritious and helps in stopping diarrhea. It's recommended not to eat large amounts in one go and not to eat Brown rice that contains fiber. There are many kinds of rice and dishes that can be made with it (please note – not to spicy!). Even cooking doesn't need to deter you – there is a special Chinese pot that makes it particularly easy. You can put the rice together with chicken or fish and thereby enrich the taste. This dish is forbidden for those who choose the Specific Carbohydrate Diet (see below).

---

[21] Lactose – the sugar that is found in milk – www.answers.com/lactose

Millet and quinoa

Millet and quinoa are grains that have a high nutritional value. Millet is particularly rich in iron, while quinoa is rich in carbohydrates and proteins. Both are very rich in vitamins. They are very easy to digest and can form a good basis for a menu for anyone who suffers from a sensitive digestive system. Millet and quinoa are also easy to cook (simple cooking with water, similar to rice, only without the need to be exact with amounts and time). They are now available not only in health shops. This dish is forbidden for those who choose the Specific Carbohydrate Diet (see below).

Organic or not organic – that is the question

The organic food faithful can skip this paragraph. For those who don't know about it, and before taking any decision as to whether to consume it or not, it's recommended that you at least learn about the advantages of organic food. The price of organic food is higher than for regular food, but the advantages are proportionately greater. Here are a number of points that as patients you should know:

Vegetables and fruit – No sprays harmful to health are used in the growing of organic vegetables and fruit, as opposed to that of regular crop growing. While it's frustrating, it's still important to know that when we consume regular vegetables and fruit, and pat ourselves on the back, aside from vitamins we are also putting harmful substances into our bodies. In our case, these substances are likely to promote inflammation. Apart from the risk, it's important to know that the nutritional value of organic fruit and vegetables is higher, and mostly, their taste is richer too.

Meat and chicken – The conventional raising of cattle and chickens also suffers from methods that serve up to our tables products filled with harmful substances such as various drugs, antibiotics and other matters. These are intended to fatten the animals and grow them to dimensions beyond their natural size. If the danger of these substances reaching your table doesn't convince you, perhaps the moral argument will (even if you aren't vegetarian) – during the process of raising the animals, the conventional chicken and meat industry causes dreadful suffering to the them, from force-feeding to slaughter. The organic industry, in its more natural approach, causes a lot less suffering in terms of this.

Fish – There are two kinds of fish: marine fish, and farmed fish. As I have mentioned, marine fish are preferable, in both taste and quality, for one simple reason – the non-interference in the raising process. (In the farm ponds they use various substances to feed the fish.)

Milk – There are those who claim that cow's milk is less healthy because of the antibiotics and drugs with which the cows are injected. Goat's milk, which contains fewer harmful substances, is therefore recommended.

I am not a fanatic about organic food, but I definitely do my best to consume it as much as I can. For those who don't consume organic food, either for economic reasons or because they don't know about its advantages, I recommend at least broadening your information on the issue, and to try out and include organic products out on your weekly menu.

Vegetables in forms you did not know

Vegetables can cause problems because of the fibers which make them up. Foods which contain fibers may scratch the interior of the bowel and cause pain and feelings of discomfort. Having said that, integrating vegetables into your daily menu is very important, mainly because of the vitamins they contain. Here are some ways to consume vegetables in a manner that makes it easier for patients who suffer from inflammation of the digestive system.

Eat little – Few people who have a sensitive bowel are able to eat a large salad and not feel that they are going to explode immediately afterwards. Therefore, if you are not prepared to give up fresh vegetables add a different vegetable each time to your meal. When it comes to dressings, incidentally, it's worth giving them up completely. It's possible to make do with a little olive oil.

Preferably cooked or steamed – Cooked or steamed vegetables are very easy to digest, and they still maintain a nutritional value similar to that of fresh vegetables. The taste may not suit everyone, but whoever can adapt and persist with it will reap great benefits for their health. It's desirable to try different forms of cooking and steaming – the investment will pay off. If you can't eat cooked vegetables, it's desirable that from time to time you have a soup that is rich in vegetables (without soup powder and with some chicken to improve the taste).

Spraying – Most vegetables are sprayed with substances that kill not only harmful organisms, but us as well. It's very important to wash vegetables thoroughly. Getting rid of the peel can help to a degree, as well as ease the digestive process. For those who are willing to make the effort, it's recommended to move to organic vegetables.

Vegetable juices – This is a fantastic way of supplying the body with the vitamins that go to make up vegetables. There are quality appliances that are made especially to separate the juice from the fiber and enable you to gulp down juice that is pure health. It's important to drink the juice soon after preparing it to take advantage of its full nutritional value. Chef's recommendation: carrot juice with a little beetroot that provides lots of iron.

Not recommended – certain vegetables that are considered acidic such as tomatoes, eggplants and peppers.

Fruit

As with vegetables, eating fruit is important mainly because of the vitamins, but is dangerous because of the fiber. Citrus fruit, for example, is completely out of the question in this regard. Here too an appropriate solution is to drink home-made juices that do not contain fiber and maintain the nutritional value of the fruit (for example those that have been squeezed in machines that filter out the fiber). If you're having fruit, do your best to eat those that are less acidic and that contain less fiber.

Dietary fiber [22]

Dietary fiber is that part of the plant that the body does not digest. It arrives at the large intestine where it is fermented by bacteria. Dietary fiber has no nutritional value and lacks calories, and therefore provides no energy at all. It's possible to distinguish between two main groups of fiber: the insoluble and the soluble.

Insoluble fiber has an outstanding capacity to absorb water, and thus increase the volume of the feces and facilitate their exit. It also limits the mobility of the intestine, shortens the time taken for the passage of food through it and exerts pressure on its walls. It's therefore clear that patients who suffer from Crohn's disease or patients who suffer from narrowing with a background of intestinal scarring must exclude this fiber from their menu.

---

[22] Nutritional fiber: www.webmd.com/diet/fiber-health-benefits-11/insoluble-soluble-fiber

Foods rich in insoluble fiber:

- Vegetables: cabbage, cauliflower, broccoli , celery, kohlrabi, peels of fruit and vegetables
- Whole grains: brown rice, whole wheat, bran, corn
- Seeds: walnuts, almonds and peanuts

Soluble fiber, as opposed to these, inhibit decomposition and the passage of food through the digestive system, and extend the feeling of fullness. They are able to absorb toxins, excess bile, cholesterol, carcinogenic substances, and even remove them from the body. They also slow down the absorption of sugar in the blood.

Foods rich in soluble fiber:

- Fruit: apples, bananas, pears
- Vegetables: zucchini, carrots, pumpkin
- Pulses: chick peas, lentils, dried beans, dried peas, broad beans and soya beans.
- Oats

Dishes rich in fiber such as fruit and vegetables, contain soluble and insoluble fiber in varying proportions. It is therefore advisable to avoid all fiber-rich foods when there is active inflammation, and to try to include them in your daily menu later on if the inflammation allows it.

Pre- and Probiotics [23]

In the digestive system there are friendly bacteria that inhibit the action of undesirable microorganisms, and that improve the breakdown of food and its digestion. These are called probiotic bacteria. There are several types of probiotic bacteria, and each part

---

[23] Probiotics: www.webmd.com/digestive-disorders/tc/probiotics-topic-overview

of the digestive system has its own different types that are capable of existing in it. During antibiotic treatment, and even after it, these positive bacteria can be harmed. They are also likely to be harmed in cases of preparation for a colonoscopy, operations on the digestive system, and frequent diarrhea and vomiting among other things. Today there are two main approaches in maintaining a balance in positive bacteria:

The first is the probiotic approach – the consumption of a food supplement or food that contains live microorganisms (usually bacteria) that have a positive action and ability to break down food. Yoghurt is an example of a food that is rich in positive bacteria. It is important to match the food or the supplement to the area of the digestive system that we want to strengthen – that they contain the same type of probiotic bacteria. The problem with this approach is that most of these bacteria do not survive the acidity of the stomach. Therefore, in order that a certain amount will reach the areas (such as the bowel) that need them, you need a large amount of bacteria.

The second approach is the prebiotic approach – the consumption of food or supplements that contain ingredients that are not digested, such as dietary fiber, that encourage the growth and thriving of friendly bacteria in the bowel.

There is research that points to probiotic bacteria aiding in maintaining remission in Colitis. There is no evidence that these bacteria directly help in suppressing Crohn's disease, but it is important to maintain them at proper levels. This is because their positive action is essential to the proper functioning of the digestive system. Because dietary fiber is not desirable for those with a sensitive bowel, you should adopt the first approach and consume food that is rich in bacteria such as yoghurt (preferably made from goat's milk) on a daily basis to maintain normal numbers of the bacteria.

Snacks and munches

This is a subject that hurts. One of the most difficult things is giving up snacks and munches when you're watching a game on TV, or giving up popcorn at a movie. Experience shows that there is no option. None of these snacks contributes to your general condition and can even mean the beginning of the next attack. The reason apparently lies in the fact that most of them are saturated with oil or that they are not made with nutritious ingredients (particularly in the case of snacks). If you cannot manage, and sometimes slide into sin, it's preferable to deal with baked snacks like pretzels, with as little oil and spices as possible.

Dried fruit

I have often been urged to eat dates and figs with the claim that they have a high nutritional value and that they have energy-giving natural sugars. Even one of the Chinese therapists that I had recommended dates, that according to him could suppress the inflammation. After I chose to begin the Specific Carbohydrate Diet I discovered dates as a source of energy and as a good substitute for sweet foods that contain sugar.

Sweets

The sweeter and more complex a food is, the more problems it causes. This is particularly true with heavy cakes that contain cow's milk, white sugar and other ingredients that can stimulate the inflammation. As one who doesn't like sweet tastes it was not especially difficult for me to give these things up. I'm sure it's not at all that easy for many others. Despite the difficulties, however, it's desirable to reduce your consumption of sweet foods as much as you can and to check out a graduated system of smaller and smaller helpings of those that are digested properly as well as those that are not. Remember that your health comes first.

Bread and pasta

Most bowel patients who take all forbidden items off the menu are usually left with bread as the main component. There are many kinds of bread. The simplest is white bread. Every alternative therapist will tell you just how bad it is, and just how much it promotes inflammation. I'm not at all sure that many patients will agree with this statement, but in any event it worth checking it yourself. The main alternative to white bread is whole meal bread. This bread is problematic for us, of course, because of the large amount of fiber that it contains. You should therefore try any other type of bread that doesn't contain a large amount of fiber on the one hand, but is not white on the other, such as spelt bread (you can find spelt in health food stores – baking bread is an experience that even people who are not ill appreciate). With every bread purchase it's advisable to pay attention to the ingredients: Sometimes what seems like whole meal bread or spelt bread can in fact contain white flour mixed with buckwheat. I'd like to add that for sensitive people it's advisable to eat the bread as toast to make it easier on the digestive system. By the same token, pasta that is not made from white flour is also recommended. Pasta can indeed be a good source of energy, but the quality of the pasta is also important to ensure easy digestion. For those who choose the Specific Carbohydrate Diet (see below), this food is not permitted.

Sugar

The claim is that white sugar is not healthy because it is processed. Various nutritionists even claim that it promotes inflammation, although this has not been proven in research. In any event it won't hurt to move to brown sugar (real, and not the "colored" kind that is offered in most coffee shops). In addition, there are natural candies that make use of sugar substitutes such as stevia (which doesn't sweeten enough to my taste), or molasses, an extract of sugar cane, and with the value of pure gold. The substitute that I prefer is honey.

Tea or coffee

Generally it's preferable to drink hot drinks rather than cold. Herbal tea is preferable to coffee, which contains caffeine, and for most, also milk – especially if it's a caffeine-free infusion which helps to calm the stomach. Anyone who is prepared to go beyond the sachets, can buy the loose herbs for infusing, or can grow them themselves in pots. A recommended infusion is from the chamomile plant, which in high concentrations is a great help in calming the digestive system.

Cola

In the past I used to drink nothing less than a liter and a half of cola a day. It was difficult for me to admit the distressing fact that I was addicted. I wouldn't be telling you anything new if I detailed here the harm that is likely to be caused to any person by the acidity, the caffeine, the sugar and the rest of ingredients that are to be found in this wonderful and cursed drink. Even from my addicted perspective cola has the most problematic characteristics. Patients with a sensitive digestive system who constantly drink cola find it particularly difficult to be rehabilitated because cola is an available source of energy, tasty, and comfortable mainly during periods of diarrhea. Heavy diarrhea causes exhaustion, and patients will seek easy sources to supplement the energy they lose. In cases like this, cola is a very bad solution. Only after you've stopped for some while do you understand just how much your stomach has not been calm, and how easy it is to develop a dependency on the amount of sugar that there is in cola. The perfect solution would of course be to move to water, although for people who are addicted (there is no easier word) as I was, the change can likely to be too sudden. Begin perhaps with raspberry juice – it also contains sugar but it is not acidic and does not contain caffeine. In any event, during times of diarrhea it's important to increase the amount you drink so that you do not become dehydrated.

Alcohol

Alcohol is not recommended for patients with inflammatory bowel disease. For those who nevertheless choose to drink, it's preferable not to drink cheap drinks, or those that are too harsh. High percentages of alcohol are likely to stimulate anyone's digestive system. It's desirable, therefore, to be careful.

Powders and ready meals

As I've mentioned, our disease is not for lazy people. In order to get quality products that don't come already prepared in packages needs time and effort. You should just stay away from the different powders of soups and meals, and from every food that comes ready from the supermarket (all the various frozen schnitzels). Apart from the fact that fresh food is both healthier and tastier, you can't exactly know what a ready meal contains. Don't be lazy – it will pay off in the future. Every minute you save with the help of ready meals will cost you an hour in the bathroom.

Pomegranate juice

Pomegranates are rich in iron, and without the seeds they are also relatively easy to digest (if a little acidic). I warmly recommend organic pomegranate juice that is a hundred percent pomegranate. It's an excellent daily nutritional supplement, especially for patients who suffer from a lack of iron. You can find the juice at organic stores throughout the year. Those who are sensitive to the acidity can dilute the juice with a little water. In the last few years pomegranate juice has been found to have anti-inflammatory properties, and hence has the capacity to help those who suffer from chronic inflammation to cope with their disease.

Supplements and additives

In cases where the food is not absorbed as it should be the attending doctor might recommend food supplements. Food supplements are important in restoring to the body what it lacks in vitamins and minerals, even those that don't appear in blood tests. Only if we balance the body nutritionally can we help it to better fight the inflammation. It's important to consume only those products that the doctor has recommended, and not to be tempted by the various supplements that are not suited to the intestines of Crohn's patients. It's important to note that the supplements that we don't consume don't cause stomach pains or deterioration of the inflammation. And be sure to check that they are indeed absorbed properly. It is important to match the supplement you're getting with the current state of the inflammation. A supplement suited to a state of calm, can cause problems with a state of active inflammation. In severe cases in which the patient does not manage to achieve nutritional balance, it's possible to give nutritional support with an enteral feeding regimen. An enteral feeding regimen means balancing by means of broken-down food constituents.

Enteral feeding formulas are divided into protein and fat constituents. Research has shown that enteral feeding is efficient in inducing remission in Crohn's in fifty to seventy percent of active flare-up cases [24]. In cases where the patient's bowel does not function, the digestive system is bypassed by means of an intravenous infusion that supplies the nutritional constituents that the patient needs. As you might expect, this method brings with it serious side-effects, and is recommended only in extreme cases.

---

[24] "Ten years" experience with an elemental diet in the management of Crohn's disease. K Teahon, I Bjarnason, M Pearson, and A J Levi – www.pubmedcentral.nih.gov/articlerender.fcgi?artid=1378738

Guidelines for the chef

Forbidden ingredients:

- Hot foods or foods that have too many spices
- Reduce fiber-rich food such as vegetables and fruit. You can use them in combination in low doses
- Brown rice and bread that contains fiber
- Beef that is difficult to digest
- Any low-quality food such as preservatives, food colorants, powders and ready foods
- Fried foods rich in oils
- Reduce cow's milk products
- Reduce foods rich in pulses such as chick-peas and beans. You can use them in combination in low doses
- Reduce eggplants and peppers
- Reduce the use of hard cheeses in order to ease digestion
- Reduce sweet foods and sugar

Permitted ingredients:

- Baked or cooked foods
- Cooked vegetables
- Eggs – organic is preferable
- Chicken – not in large amounts
- Fish – not in large amounts
- Goat's milk, goat's milk yoghurt and soft cheeses
- Honey

The following ingredients are allowed but are not part of the Specific Carbohydrate Diet:

- Fruit and vegetables that are low in fiber such as sweet potato, garlic, pumpkin, zucchini, artichokes, carrots, potato and more
- Bread and pasta – recommended, but only if made with flour that is not white such as spelt
- White rice
- Root vegetables
- Soya

In addition to your current diet it's important keep up a constant monitoring according to various parameters to ensure that there is no suspicion of malnutrition. With children it is especially important to monitor height and weight. You need to do blood tests in order to identify nutritional deficiencies, especially of iron and vitamin B12, and to bring their levels up with food supplements, injections or transfusions when necessary. Balancing the diet for a Crohn's or Colitis patient is not a simple matter. Even with mentoring (which doesn't exist for most people) it is difficult to balance the digestive system, especially in the case of active inflammation. However, it is important to remember that the hard work pays off. A patient in the right nutritional state will deal better with the inflammation, experience fewer difficulties in daily activities, and will maintain a normal bodily condition. You should take your diet as seriously as a prescription medication – a correct diet is your real medication.

The Specific Carbohydrate Diet – SCD

The Specific Carbohydrate Diet or SCD is aimed at patients with inflammatory bowel diseases, those diseases affects the intestinal wall, and as a result of which the bowel has difficulties in breaking down disaccharides and multi-saccharides that remain in the bowel and comprise a substrate in which bacteria grow and cause additional harm to the intestine.

The diet was developed by Elaine Gottschall, a clinical dietician and bio-chemist whose daughter was diagnosed as a Colitis patient. Despite intensive drug treatment her condition deteriorated until Elaine moved her to the Specific Carbohydrate Diet. Within two years the symptoms from which the girl had suffered disappeared. After a few years she returned to a normal diet and her health continued to be excellent. Following that, Elaine researched the diet and published her results in a book *Breaking the Vicious Cycle*.

Many patients have said that the diet has helped them, although the research results are not definitive for all patients. The diet is not an easy one, but patients who have achieved a state of calmness have returned to a normal diet after a few years.

With this method you need to avoid foods that contain disaccharides and multi-saccharides, which means that you can't eat foods that contain the flour of any grain whatsoever – corn, potato, sugar, rice, chick-peas, pulses, soya and more. You are allowed to eat the following: honey, eggs, fruit and vegetables, meat, chicken and fish and types of nuts (you can for example prepare cakes with almond or walnut flour).

You can find the full list of what products are allowed and what are not on the internet. The name of the book is *Breaking the Vicious Cycle. The Specific Carbohydrate Diet, by Elaine Gottschall.* The site is www.breakingtheviciouscycle.info

.

Medical Cannabis

If I had to tell you that if you spread a little of a certain powder on your tongue it would help calm your pain, wouldn't you try it? You would certainly ask me what the side-effects are. If you don't go over the recommended dose, the side-effects are negligible, certainly relative to other medication. There could be a little tiredness which passes with time, and merriment – a feeling of happiness and laughter without obvious reason. In addition there is an increase in appetite. There are other side effects with prolonged use. You should always consult with the doctor and the supplier before use.

Despite these side effects, this powder can improve the state of the inflammation. Researchers have found that patients report a significant improvement in their inflammation and their general feeling after using cannabis.

The first time I tried cannabis I had been living with Crohn's for sixteen years. I went through all the dubious experiences that this disease can offer: pain, diarrhea, and one serious operation.

I had already tried all the solutions that western medicine has to offer, and I still didn't feel well. In fact, I felt bad, even very bad. Endless diarrhea, and frequent pain that wouldn't pass for weeks. I would go around for whole days at a time with permanent pain, like a static noise that won't go away.

I researched the subject of cannabis and I found that many patients with various diseases use this drug. Until the nineteenth century, cannabis was legal as a natural medication for the relief of pain. Today many patients use cannabis on a regular basis to cope better with their health problems, and live a normal life. In a conversation that I had with one of the suppliers of medical cannabis it turned out that the age range of the patients was very wide. From adults who use cannabis to sleep to children who receive drops that help them to overcome, for example, the feelings of nausea after chemotherapy. Patients who consume cannabis on a permanent basis do not feel the side effects of dizziness and feelings of floating that go with its first use and succeed in functioning at various forms of work.

As with many other treatments, cannabis needs to be matched with the patient. Patients need to go through structured guidance from a qualified person and to invest effort in finding the dose that suits them and in seeking the supplier that will allow them to obtain the medication in a form that suits them: as a powder, as drops or as leaves for smoking.

After a great deal of effort, I managed to obtain permission for a monthly dose of cannabis, and I went through guidance on how to use it. I understood that it is important to relate to cannabis as medication and to pay attention to the dosages, otherwise there could be side effects, some of which are serious. In my first attempts to smoke the cannabis, I choked, and I didn't feel anything – certainly not an improvement in my pain or inflammation. After a few days I had taken too much, and my head spun terribly. I decided to take just a few puffs before sleep, but I still didn't feel any improvement. After a few weeks I abandoned it. I felt that cannabis was another area which only provides hope without any real results.

It was only after a few months that I returned to reading about the subject on the internet. I understood that I had made the classic mistake of thinking it was a wonder drug. In my innocence I had thought that it was enough to take a few puffs of a cigarette that I didn't know the composition of, and I would feel better.

I discovered that medicinal cannabis is classified into two main groups: Sativa and Indica. The two types contain differing amounts of THC, the active ingredient that provides most of the medical effects of the plant. Both cannabis types are therefore effective in treating various problems.

- Sativa has a stimulating and energetic effect. It particularly affects the nervous system and the brain, and is especially suited to reducing depression and nausea, increasing appetite and reducing pain.
- Indica calms pain and induces sleep. It is therefore recommended that you use it in the evening or before sleep. It is Indica that helps in reducing pain, with sleeping. It helps by making it easier when there is a state of inflammation, reducing stress and anxiety, easing feelings of nausea and headaches, and it increases appetite. It is thus particularly suitable in the treatment of diseases like Crohn's or Colitis.

It is Indica that helps maintain continuous sleep even when there is pain. It significantly helps improve physical condition during periods of pain in which it is difficult to get any sleep at all, certainly not quality and continuous sleep.

Different suppliers of medicinal cannabis sell various kinds composed of differing percentages of Indica and Sativa. Mostly they use simple names such as "day" or "night", or they use colors to differentiate them. In addition those who sell cannabis don't always know the exact proportions of the mixture that reaches the patient. It is therefore important to find a supplier who knows how to supply the relevant amount and that the medicinal cannabis that he is selling is from the Indica strain and is of sufficient level and quality.

In addition I discovered that you don't have to smoke cannabis. You can consume it as a powder or as drops that have the power to bring about the same effect, but this too varies from patient to patient.

I eventually found a quality supplier who also knew how to provide answers and explain in detail the medicinal use of cannabis, as opposed to other suppliers who relate to the matter as if they were selling vegetables. During periods of pain I use cannabis before sleep by taking two puffs of a mixture that contains mainly the Indica strain. Sometimes during the day I use the powder that I sprinkle into hot tea or over food, and it helps to ease the pain.

It's not something that happened in just a day or two, but bit by bit something calmed down and I began to sleep much better. My appetite improved, and the pains passed. I used cannabis for a year, in addition to conventional medicine. During this time my condition improved and I didn't experience any serious attacks.

From the side effects point of view, it was difficult at first to breathe the smoke in. After that the sense of floating and of dizziness was problematic, but with time it passed – especially when I don't go over the correct dose.

As with many areas of this disease, if you relate to it as a curiosity and a joke or as something cool that is worth trying, the results will turn out accordingly. However, if you relate to it in a serious way and you really try to discover if it can help, and what the right dose is for you, it can significantly improve the state of your health.

Obtaining permission

During the period when I felt ill and all the medical tests showed that the situation was not good, I reported to various doctors about it. Not even one doctor thought about recommending this drug. More than that, after I understood that in fact there were not many treatments left that I had not yet tried in order to feel better, and that cannabis could help me deal at least with the pain, many doctors were not prepared to give me permission. It is something that to this day I still do not understand. A person was standing before them who was suffering, and they had no solution to his problem (in fact they did have a number of solutions – that didn't work, and with horrendous side-effects). I am employed in structured work, a father to four children, and it's clear that I wasn't looking to start a cannabis celebration, and still, when it came to asking permission for a drug that does no harm and can even help, I came up against a wall of ethics on the part of most of the doctors. While it's true that there is a concern that ninety-nine people in a hundred who request permission to use cannabis, have no medical problem, this is not a reason to prevent the one patient who does suffer, from getting even the smallest chance of reducing their pain – a chance that would allow us to have a normal life. I hope that many more doctors will know how to recognize the patients who do need this medicine, and will not pile on obstacles in addition to the disease.

Clinical research

During clinical research [25] that was conducted for eight weeks at Meir Hospital in Kfar Saba in Israel, two groups were examined: In the first group there were patients who for three years had received cannabis cigarettes, and in the second group there were patients who had received cigarettes containing a placebo. Among twenty-one out of the thirty patients who used cannabis, there was a significant improvement after use. The need for other medication was significantly reduced. Before the use of cannabis fifteen of the patients had nineteen operations over an average period of nine years, and after three years of cannabis use, only two patients required surgery.

---

[25] www.norml.org/news/2011/09/22/study-crohn-s-patients-who-use-cannabis-report-fewer-surgeries-are-less-likely-to-use-prescription-drugs

A mother's words

One of the things that is most difficult for every mother, and in my case, a mother of a Crohn's disease patient, is the mere knowledge that your child is suffering. On a practical level I immediately prepared myself to find ways to improve the quality of his life: every item of processed food, every bottle of sweetened drink, snacks and every other thing that could be thought of as problematic for digestion was immediately thrown out of the house. The kitchen was converted into a natural kitchen that included cooked and fresh food on a daily basis in accordance with Rafael's preferences. The new menu included fresh fish, fresh bread, eggs, tuna, homemade hummus, honey, steamed vegetables etc. It wasn't easy. The experiment in dragging the entire house into a change was truly problematic, although only for a short period. In the long term we all got used to it, and even profited from it.

The internalization of the change of set-up in the house, and alongside that the internalization that you have an ill child, has to occur as quickly as possible, in order to help both the child and oneself as the parent. More than that it is very hard, almost impossible, to pass on the message of change to the child, without including all the members of the household (it's important to speak to the siblings and to explain the situation to them).

The frequent stomach pains, the ongoing suffering, the diarrhea, the skin irritations and the weakness – all these brought us to an understanding that a change of diet would not be enough. We thus checked every alternative treatment that was recommended. In my experience one should never rule out any treatment channel. One can always find a treatment that will improve the situation, whether it's a local massage, conversations and encouragements that will increase the child's belief and motivation, or whether it's Chinese acupuncture, garlic or herbal essences. It is of course important to reduce the level of stress at home, even if it means reducing the hours of work of one of the parents – from this point of view it's desirable that there is always someone at home; and yes, it's important to talk – and lots.

Another important issue is the importance of physical activity despite the general weakness of the child. Here, it is sometimes necessary for the parents to act against their initial instincts and to encourage activities such as these: when Rafael decided that he wanted to go on a diving course, my first response was to refuse. My husband convinced me to agree and we began to prepare for the course. We explained to the friend with whom he went to the course about Rafael's condition, the need to maintain his routines of continuous eating (and in small portions) throughout the day. For this mission we procured a backpack full of sandwiches and drinks. The benefit that Rafael got from the course and ourselves along with him, was beyond our expectations. His success on the course strengthened his confidence, and increased his understanding that there was nothing that he could not do. There is no doubt that physical activity helps and strengthens the state of mind and without question there is nothing more important than this.

I will not deny that there were times of despair, a feeling of helplessness from the inability to help the child in his pain, the diarrhea and his struggle with the various tests. However, one always needs to remember that we, the parents, are an anchor for the children at every age. It is therefore important that the message that we transmit is calm and by no account hysterical. Stress does not heal the disease – on the contrary.

Apart from that it's important to maintain a supporting environment of friends – even when Rafael was receiving treatment at home we also ensured that his friends would be there to help him to get through the hard times. The direct connection between emotional and mental overload and stomach pain is indisputable. One therefore has to be aware, and to respond accordingly and immediately. The basic conditions for lots of structured sleep, healthy food and calm surroundings contribute to improvement of the daily quality of life.

In conclusion, and briefly – a little professional information. As an aromatherapist [26] (aromatherapy is the massage and application of essential oils on the skin to ease and heal it during periods of irritation, pain or stress) I immediately took out all my tools of treatment in order to ease my son's condition. Crohn's disease is a disease of deficiencies which can cause, among other things, damage and a lack of vitality to hair in the long term. A mixture of oils in a scalp massage brings about improvement in oxygenation and a better nutrition for the hair. Therefore when there is irritation, burns or rashes, especially because of the frequent diarrhea, it's desirable to use a mixture of oils that heal the skin such as jojoba, rose-hip, evening primrose, vitamin E with lavender and Roman chamomile. Tepid baths are also recommended as they calm rashes and the patient himself. One can of course always combine suitable aromatherapy oils with various treatments such as reflexology which can ease stomach pain and reduce the level of stress.

---

[26] Aromatherapy: The use of essential and base oils to treat body and soul

Alternative Medicine

In this chapter I will focus on two areas of alternative medicine, areas which in my experience have it within their capacity to help Crohn's and Colitis patients. The sources of the information that appears here are leading professionals in the field. The aim is to present these areas in a thorough way that will deepen your knowledge of the treatment methods and with the world-view behind them. I believe that a thorough familiarity with these areas will help you in choosing the treatment that suits you on the way to a calmer and healthier period in your life.

Chinese medicine and Crohn's disease

This information is based on an interview with Itzik Emmanuel Zangi, a graduate of the Alternative Medical College and the University of Zhejiang in China, lecturer in ancient Chinese writings, director of clinics in the central and Jerusalem regions of Israel, treating chronic inflammatory diseases by means of medicinal herbs, acupuncture and Tui Na.

Chinese medicine – general principles and differences from other fields of alternative treatment

Chinese medicine was developed by trial and error a few thousand years ago. The central idea consists of looking at processes in nature and comparing them with processes in people that are viewed as an inseparable part of nature. When a person does not live in harmony with nature it may create a lack of balance that brings disease. Therefore, in order to avoid disease you must listen to nature and its dictates. This listening may be expressed by wearing warm clothes when it gets cold, sleeping during the hours of darkness and not during the day, paying attention to inner feelings, avoiding repressing things, frustration, anger, and any similar obsessive feelings. Chinese medicine is fundamentally a preventative medicine. A healthy lifestyle, nutrition and bodily care are therefore extremely important – and all of it, as I have mentioned, is in order to avoid a lack of balance.

Even if there is a lack of balance, Chinese medicine can provide a solution: being a holistic medicine Chinese medicine relates to the person as a complete system divided into sub-systems which are interconnected. This is the reason for the belief according to which a lack of balance causes damage to the entire system, and not just in one organ or tissue. The idea is to find the root of the problem, which might well not be in the damaged organ, but in another distressed organ – this would then be the organ in which effort will be invested. This approach might explain the failure of conventional medicine in cases in which the disease breaks out and reappears, despite surgical intervention.

Treatment tools in Chinese medicine

An exact diagnosis precedes Chinese medical treatment (usually via a check of the tongue and pulse and questions). The more accurate the diagnosis the more efficient the treatment. The treatment is accomplished with the use of herbal remedies, acupuncture, Moxa and Tui Na (Chinese physiotherapy). Combined with this are preventative and healing exercises such as Tai Ch'i, Qigong, correct diet and lifestyle.

The unique characteristics of Chinese medicine

Today Chinese medicine occupies a significant place in the world of alternative medicine. Compared with other treatment methods, its uniqueness lies in an exact matching of patient and treatment. The causes of disease vary from patient to patient, and hence there might well be different treatments for different patients with the same disease. This is because of the principle of balance which is the basis of Chinese medicine and the differences between patients.

The efficacy of Chinese medicine is recognizable in the combination of several treatment techniques, among them acupuncture, the use of herbs and even physiotherapy (also for internal problems). The result is a treatment of great capacity and power that works on a number of levels at the same time and which is matched to the condition of the patient. The relatively short and simple diagnoses together with the fact that it is possible to begin the treatment at any stage of the disease, bring great advantages to this system. If that were not enough, the fact that it relates to the general lack of balance in the body can prevent a deterioration in health in areas not connected with the patient's disease.

Chinese medicine and Crohn's disease

In the ancient books that deal with Chinese medicine, there are references to bowel disease under the complimentary category "diseases of many diarrheas" or "watery diarrhea". There are references to additional symptoms that are unique to Crohn's disease, among them bleeding, inflammation and more. The books detail in a very exact way what the conditions are that can cause this disease, and here are some representative examples:

Chinese medicine accurately diagnoses the type of diarrhea, for example it deals with issues in the development of diarrhea against a background of cold or heat: "cold" diarrhea is characterized by stomach pains and feces that contain undigested food, while "hot" diarrhea has a sharp smell accompanied by burning and sometimes even bleeding and pus. The treatment for these two conditions will be completely different, even though both might be diagnosed as Crohn's disease. Another example has to do with spleen function. In the view of Chinese medicine, the spleen is responsible for the breakdown and transporting of food. Accordingly, weakness in the spleen that is caused by, among other things, unsuitable (cold, fatty, heavy) food, is likely to be the foundation for the development of mucus that itself can create pus and inflammation.

Therefore, in order to accurately diagnose the disease, it is necessary to relate to the influence of particular organs that occupy an important place, and are a central cause, in the development of the disease: the liver, the gall bladder and the heart. As opposed to conventional western medicine, Chinese medicine sees the functioning of these organs as hugely important in the development of the disease because these organs connect the disease to mental function ("emotional background"). Emmanuel is of the opinion that these organs are integrally involved in the development of various stages of the disease, and that emotions such as tension, anger and frustration, create a disturbance in the energy of the liver or the heart and have an influence on the digestive system by means of the connections between the organs.

Main methods of treatment

Treatment for Crohn's in Chinese medicine is separated into treatment for acute conditions and treatment for chronic conditions. The aim of the acute condition treatment is the calming of the attacks of pain, stopping the bleeding and improving the condition of the inflammation. The aim in the chronic treatment is to balance the basic tendencies of the body that have brought on the disease. For both these approaches both herbs and acupuncture may be used.

Acupuncture points on the meridians [27] affect the relevant organ or organs and bring about balance. From this point of view, the use of herbs is very efficient, as much scientific research has proven. Every herb has specific qualities vis-à-vis heat and cold, the organs on which they have an effect and which they strengthen, an ability to promote blood-flow, the breakdown of mucus, the calming of the mind and so on. The herbs are personally matched to every patient according to the diagnosis of the disease.

An additional treatment technique is heating by means of Moxa. Heat treatment has been known for thousands of years and many qualities have been attributed to it. The world-view behind this technique is that the origin of many diseases is cold that penetrates the body. The cold drains to a particular place and creates various disturbances. This technique uses a particular strain of the sage plant to heat a certain area of the body, mainly the navel. It is customary to treat problems relating to moisture and to strengthen the immune system by heating this area. In this way it reaches the disease directly.

The required goals

The main goal is of course to reach a state of remission in the disease: inactive inflammation, freedom from pain, and proper functioning of the bowel. It's important to remember that frequent diarrhea, not to mention bleeding, demand a great deal of energy from the body, and stopping it is therefore essential. Only after that should you move to a more fundamental treatment for the state of inflammation.

---

[27]   Meridian – the channels, according to Chinese medicine, along which bodily energy flows.

Lifestyle and nutrition

Crohn's disease is frequently characterized by an accumulation of warm mucus and "plugs" of blood. It's therefore desirable for patients to avoid first and foremost foods that produce mucus such as dairy products, fatty foods, food that is difficult to digest, cold food and alcohol. Apart from this you should avoid food that encourages bacterial activity such as sweet foods that contain sugar, yeast, etcetera. As opposed to this, orange vegetables such as pumpkin, carrot and sweet potato might strengthen the spleen. Also, recent research has proven that the consumption of camel milk is efficient in treating this disease. However, beyond the importance of diet, Emmanuel believes that there is a critical importance in a lifestyle that is free from tension and frustration. It's desirable to do physical activities, to persevere with hobbies, and with anything else that can reduce the level of mental and physical tension.

Combination with conventional treatment

It is possible and desirable to combine Chinese medical treatment with conventional western medicine. It's important to emphasize that there is no contradiction between different treatments. Data shows that in countries where they make use of both types of treatment the percentages of success are high and benefit patients greatly: Patients are not torn between two worlds and benefit much from the two treatments together. Chinese medicine seeks to balance the causes of the disease and strives to reach a general balance. The patient can therefore come to treatment in Chinese medicine at any stage of treatment, even if he has already undergone intensive conventional western procedures and used any drug at all (including steroids). An obvious disadvantage of western treatment lies in its approach of focusing only on symptoms, as opposed to Chinese treatment which, as I've mentioned, sees the body as a whole system.

More than that, the effectiveness of herbal treatment and acupuncture in overcoming the side-effects of steroid use, and in reducing the use of steroids, has long been proven.

Medical Qigong

This section is based on an interview with Dror Aloni, who has been involved with medical Qigong since 1999. Dror began his studies in the field at the Yetsira School under the leadership of Ohad Kedem, and over the years he has completed his studies to achieve the degree of Certified Guide in Qigong [28] and Tai Ch'i [29], and participated in advanced studies in workshops in Israel and abroad with various teachers and masters in the field. Aside from this, Dror, since finishing his studies as an industrial engineer at the Technion in Haifa, serves as organizational adviser at the Seker company. From when he was ten years old Dror has struggled with a rare cancer. He has done this with the aid of a range of conventional treatments (bone marrow transplants, chemotherapy, radiation, operations and radioactive treatments) combined with alternative treatments (Qigong, Tai Ch'I, guided imagery, meditation, medicinal herbs, acupuncture and healing). Over the years Dror delved into the unique medical path of medical Qigong, and other alternative treatments over a range of different diseases (particularly cancer). He also dealt with improving the ability to cope with the intensive treatments that he endured.

---

[28] Qigong or Ch'I Kung – an ancient Chinese movement art

[29] Tai Ch'I, or in its full name, Tai Ch'IChuan – a Chinese martial art of the Kung Fu family

Basic principles of traditional Chinese medicine

The ancient Chinese approach explains medical principles by dividing various alternative dimensions into three classes: The physical dimension, the energy dimension and the spiritual dimension of human tissue. Any effect on one or more of these dimensions necessarily brings a change to the others. In this way a complex system is created whereby the diagnosis and the treatment behave in a non-linear and asymmetrical way. This means that you cannot necessarily measure or analyze the progress or deterioration of any one factor without taking into account the progress or deterioration of others that create together with it a multi-dimensional matrix. It is almost impossible to measure this matrix with the knowledge and tools that exist today. It is exactly for this reason that the holistic "complete" approach was developed in China (and even before that, in India), an approach that maintains that it is possible to construct and analyze the full picture placed before us, not by dividing it into the smallest pieces that make it up, but rather by accepting the picture itself as a whole that we do not have the capacity to divide.

The philosophical principle that stands at the center of the issues I have spoken about here, actually reflects the essence of the conflict between Western and Chinese medicine. While in Western medicine extraordinary effort and millions of dollars are invested to thoroughly research human tissue by means of dividing it into cells, genes, proteins, molecules and so on, in Chinese medicine they work on the development of the physical, energy and spiritual capacities of diagnosis and treatment of the person as a single entity. These two approaches have given birth to two totally different models of looking at the same phenomenon that is "the person", or in the wider sense, "life". For this reason a Chinese doctor is able to diagnose a lack of blood in the liver, without sending the patient for blood tests to indicate liver function. This is because the liver, according to the Chinese view, is not the liver according to the Western view. And the problem of the liver according to the former is not necessarily seen as a problem of the liver according to the latter, and vice versa. For the same reason exactly, a Western doctor might diagnose an abnormality in a patient's liver function by means of routine blood tests, and immediately give instructions for preventative treatment, while a Chinese doctor might arrive at a diagnosis that is not at all connected with the liver.

Despite this conflict it is of course possible to combine these two approaches, approaches that emanate from a basic difference in the thought processes of eastern and western people. Today with the meteoric development of the field of communication and the creation of the global village, the world has become more and more accessible for everyone, and in this regard any one approach can learn from its peers. As a result of this, an approach has thus begun to develop that combines these two different philosophies. In tandem with this, innovative approaches are being developed in the sciences generally, and in physics in particular, whose basis is the understanding that there are more similarities than differences between the philosophies of the ancient world and the theories of the future in the world of science. An example of the bridge that has been built between Chinese and western medicine can be seen in the diagnosis in Chinese medicine of a lack of blood in the kidneys. This diagnosis can be "translated" to western medicine as a reduction in kidney function that can be seen in blood tests. The Chinese and western doctors arrive at the same diagnosis, but in a different language.

The medical principles of medical Qigong exercises

The ancient principles of medical Qigong are based on the principles that I have described in the previous paragraph. Qigong is one of the five ways of treatment known to Chinese medicine, alongside therapeutic herbs, acupuncture, nutrition and touch therapy. Their combination creates a full and complete therapeutic response that stands fast against the range of problems and diseases which confronts humanity. Qigong exercises are in fact simple exercises that combine physical movement with breathing exercises (sometimes with the making of sounds) as well as exercises of imagination and awareness.

The exercises themselves are based on the model of Chinese medicine (the five elements, the Ch'i meridians on the body, etc). Each exercise works on the body and soul in different ways and is matched to the needs of the patient. The treatments have the capacity to release energy blockages, to stream ch'i to areas where there is a deficiency, to spread ch'i from areas where is there is a surplus and to return the body to perfect balance.

Western medicine recognizes the existence of much research that proves the benefits derived from Qigong exercises, and their capacity to treat various diseases. Other research still has difficulty in providing an explanation by means of western parameters, especially with regard to the working procedure during the execution of the exercises. A few of the explanations relate the benefits to changes in physiology (bone, muscle, tendons, ligaments and joints), improvement in the cardiovascular system (the heart and blood vessel system) [30], improvement in the respiratory system, improvement in the nervous system, including the brain and the spine.

Benefits relating to the action of alternative medicine and Qigong in particular

Here are a few obvious advantages that Dror relates to the action of the alternative medicine he practices, and in particular the field of medical Qigong. I must stress that the advantages are presented here on the basis of his personal experience and the knowledge he has accumulated from the literature and articles on the subject and not on scientific research. The advantages relate specifically to treatments he has experienced, although it is very easy to extrapolate from them to the treatments that Crohn's patients undergo.

---

[30] Circulatory system: The cardiovascular system, the blood or circulatory system – the system that includes the heart and blood vessels.

Speedy recovery from surgery - Throughout all the seven operations that Dror had from the age of twenty his recovery was always quicker than expected – he was never in hospital for longer than two days before being discharged. More than that, his range of movement and his stability were almost not impaired despite repeated operations on his chest cavity, armpit and throat. The pains were always at a tolerable level and he almost never needed painkillers.

Coping with radiation treatment and chemotherapy - During all the many treatments he received Dror never suffered from the many and well-known side-effects. He felt a certain tiredness but continued to function normally – he worked and studied. Therefore, and perhaps this is the most important thing of all, the cancerous cells almost always responded excellently to the treatment and disappeared after a few minimal treatments: All this, despite many treatments of different kinds that could have caused great systemic damage to Dror's body along with a minimal response of the cancer to the treatment.

Coping spiritually - During the many years that Dror coped with the disease he managed to maintain his optimism, joy of life and positive approach. It could be that this is to do with his character, although he claims, that it is without a shadow of a doubt the medical Qigong, meditation and guided imagery exercises that strengthened this approach of his and helped him to emerge easily and quickly from the difficult moments of depression and anxiety. Medical Qigong does not prevent anger or depression in dealing with difficulties, but it definitely helps you to quickly extract yourself from these situations.

Using the tools of medical Qigong to treat diseases

From what I have said in the previous paragraphs it is clear that there is no material difference between cancer and Crohn's disease if you look at the subject in a holistic and complete way. We are talking about serious and chronic diseases in which the spiritual aspect plays a leading role. This fact is completely acceptable to western doctors and is not only the heritage of alternative medicine practitioners.

Today it seems that Medical Qigong doesn't only help with coping spiritually and physically with the disease, but also generates a special motivation to immerse yourself and to investigate in a never-ending search for creative solutions. Surprisingly, or perhaps not surprisingly, this theory connects perfectly with the most widely known phenomenon in the world of alternative medicine in the field of cancer: patients who have been enlightened enough in their conquering of cancer to make a meaningful change in their lives – that is, a change for the best in the areas of work, family and so on – are precisely the patients who have confronted their cancers in the best way and survived as cancer patients for periods of time longer than had been expected. It seems that this harmony is the main reason that Medical Qigong is an efficacious treatment tool. The physical, spiritual and mental exercises bring the patient to a point at which he takes responsibility for his condition, and attempts to change it. In doing this, the teachings of Qigong are capable of bringing about a change of direction and approach to life which greatly strengthens the process of self-healing.

The second main point that greatly helps the healing process is the increase in awareness, sensitivity and listening of the patient to everything that occurs around him. Qigong exercises greatly increase these abilities, particularly in regard to physical and spiritual awareness. The accepted norms in the modern western world cause people to continue in the stressful routines of their lives, even when their bodies emphatically signal to them that they need to slow down their pace a little and rest. When a person has a fever he takes a pill and goes to work. If his back is sore, he will take another pill and continue. Heart and asthma attacks and innumerable other examples are evidence of the lack of sensitivity, awareness and often even the apathy of people when it comes to their condition. The tiny signals that the body sends out do not elicit the necessary responses. The readiness to change unfortunately comes only after crises in the form of cancer, diabetes, slipped discs, nervous breakdowns or Crohn's. As opposed to this, with the help of exercises to strengthen sensitivity to the most minute changes in the body, it is possible to identify problems at very early stages and to know how to treat them. We thus learn not to exaggerate, not to stretch our limitations into unhealthy territory, to avoid every aspect of extremism, and in general, to do what is good for us.

Before he concludes, Dror asks to emphasize an important additional view concerning the healing. In a book that he recently came across there is a beautiful sentence that speaks about the classical learning of Tai Ch'i: ***"The person who does not practice it finds it difficult to understand the depth of the writings, while the person who does practice understands them even before reading."*** That is to say: Guys – in order to experience the real depth of the wonderful capacities of Medical Qigong, it is not enough to read this chapter. In order to reach a real and deep understanding you have to practice it religiously and with dedication.

Cancer has become an inseparable part of Dror. He lives with the disease, and it lives with him. This is a fact that will probably never change, just as Medical Qigong has also become an indivisible part of him. This is without doubt 'thanks' to the cancer that returned when he was twenty. Dror claims that he cannot imagine how his life would look if the cancer had not returned and if he had not as result entered into the world of self-healing. In an almost chilling way he thanks cancer for having shown him the way to this wonderful world. Dror believes that Medical Qigong holds both his spiritual and physical body together when in similar circumstances he could have broken and collapsed already a long time ago. He chose to end his words with a special and wonderful quote of Avner Shilo, a guided imagery therapist who healed himself of cancer:

"I had the privilege and the pleasure of becoming ill with cancer and of being healed through my own efforts, completely through my own efforts."

In 2012 Dror passed away at the age of thirty-three as one of the only patients in the world who survived for a long time with active Neuroblastoma cancer from which he suffered from the age of ten. He was a friend and his way of coping with the challenges of the disease made him a hero in the eyes of everyone who had the privilege of knowing him.

Integrative Medicine
The combination of alternative and conventional medicine

This chapter is based on the book Medicine and The Seven Universal Laws by senior cardiologist and bypass surgeon Dr Nader Butto. In his book Dr Butto describes the integrative medicine model that relates to the person as a harmonious and complicated combination of body, mind, soul and spirit, and sheds a new light on the connection between mental crisis and bodily disease.

Alternative and Conventional medicine

Despite the achievements of conventional medicine in emergency and trauma medicine and in advancing public health, it has seriously failed in the treatment and the prevention of chronic diseases. Most of the diseases from which people suffer are chronic diseases. None of the new drugs and sophisticated technologies has brought about the prevention of these diseases, and more than that, there is a continuing rise in their occurrence and in the resulting mortality.

Alternative medicine relates to every treatment of body and mind whose aim is to prevent or heal disease, with methods based on the principle of combinations that bring balance between body and mind, and the soul. These methods are based, at least theoretically, on the deep connection between body, mind and soul and transfer messages of balance, naturalness and health that are created as a result of prevention of disease at the physical and mental level.

Alternative medicine provides a better answer to chronic diseases by focusing, with delicate and long-term intervention, on prevention in order to allow the healing powers of our bodies, with the aid of natural medicines, to bring about a state of healing. The disadvantage of this approach to medicine is the lack of a scientific basis to the treatment methods. There are cases where it could be that damage has been caused as a result of the neglect of conventional medicine, especially in severe cases in which conventional medicine could have helped more. There exists evidence of considerable damage associated with alternative treatments and products whose efficacy, quality and safety are not known, as well as a lack of qualification and supervision in many practitioners.

Integrative medicine – a combination of two worlds

Integrative medicine allows the practice of medicine that combines Alternative medicine with the methods of diagnosis and treatment of Conventional medicine. There is a series of techniques that can be combined in order to ease the suffering of people whose health is problematic. One should make the most of the contribution of each system individually.

Trauma and spiritual views of disease

Today it is recognized that at the base of every disease lies a range of causes. Many diseases are described as idiopathic (without explanation) – that is without clear cause, and there is no possibility of isolating one single main reason for their existence. Every disease in which a main cause can be isolated is a result of three causes:

- The biological structure and the conditions of the biological defense systems
- Psychological conflicts and types of stress response
- Environmental factors (bacteria, viruses, dietary sensitivity etc.)

The combination of biological structure and psychological type which are determined by the genetic code can give an early indication of the development of disturbances, although it's not enough that a specific phenomenon occurs. A person's genetic code causes him to behave in a particular way which brings him to experience crises of a certain type. The presence of defense factors such as the familial health environment, prevents the creation of conditions for the outbreak of disease. Biological immunity provides strength which is expressed as a more powerful resistance under threat, and which yields positive outcomes, despite conditions of heightened risk.

Pressure and stress
"In peace of the mind will be peace for the entire body"
Isaac Arama

Stress

One of the main sources of disturbances of balance in our lives, one that causes a chain reaction in all the systems, is stress. Stress has been recorded as one of the first and main reasons for disease in the modern world in which competitiveness and achievement are the fundamental values and the measure of success.

Stress is the response to a circumstance that is perceived by the mental/physical system as one of existential threat, and it can be seen also in animals in the wild. It is therefore viewed as a response of self-preservation whose purpose is to survive in dangerous situations, and which facilitates self-defense in emergencies.

According to estimates more than a hundred million people in the US suffer from continuing stress resulting in damage to the functioning of various bodily systems. The common causes of emotional stress are: work pressures, problems in relating to one's surroundings, financial difficulties and repressed negative emotions. Physiological causes of stress are chronic pain, surgery, burns, accident injury, disease and more. These situations create a physiological chain reaction that in time burdens the bodily systems beyond what they can endure.

Examples of some bodily responses to stress:

- Cramps in the digestive system
- A rise in heart rate and blood pressure
- Excessive blood clotting
- Muscle cramps

The purpose of cramps in the digestive system is to channel more blood to essential organs like the heart, lungs, brain, eyes and muscles in order to cope better with the danger.

Pressure as a positive motivator

Pressure can be a positive motivator when it appears as an acute response to a brief event. Thus, for example, during a sporting activity, the increased production of the hormone endorphin brings about an improvement in general feeling and the inhibition of negative moods. High levels of endorphin in the blood regulate the state of mind, and cause calmness, an increase in the level of awareness, a reduction in physical exhaustion and better coping with pressures in the long term.

Pressure as a negative motivator

Exposure to continuing tension and the pressure response that disturbs the hormonal balance for an extended period causes severe damage to health, and among other things, inflammation of the bowel, and a "nervous" intestine. The danger of developing autoimmune diseases also increases.

Human types and pressure

There are three facets that are connected with the type of person who suffers from stress.

The biological facet: This depends on the biological make-up of the person. It is possible to describe this facet exactly by means of a description of the genetic code.

The mental facet: This depends on the emotional intelligence of the person, his skill and experience in similar situations, in the defenses he has developed for himself, in the emotional support he receives from his environment, and in the physical data that allow him to control the situation.

The societal facet: Societal and familial connections can mitigate the impact of stress on a person. They allow him to live through the pressure and to accept it with greater ease. They give him the tools, the energy and the motivation to cope with the tension. The absence of external support – personal or material – can strengthen the source of the stress and weaken the person's ability to cope with it.

Hostility and disease

Research has found that the element of hostility is the central cause in the development of tension, and ultimately in the development of disease. The exaggerated expression of hostility is also connected with social isolation. There are three expressions of hostility – anger, cynicism and lack of belief – which cause a person to be emotionally and mentally disconnected from others, something which exposes him to bodily disease that develops against a mental background.

Optimism and pessimism

A great deal of research has shown that people who have a pessimistic interpretation of life events are less healthy, tend to depression, and turn more to general and mental health services. In contrast with them optimists enjoy a good state of health thanks to an efficient immune system, reach old age in good condition, and live longer. There is no doubt that a large part of one's approach to life is embedded in one's personality. Freedom from inhibitions and resolving rigid defense mechanisms, education from a young age and even clinical interventions, can turn an individual's personal interpretation in an optimistic direction, and consequently also his life expectancy.

Happiness

There is no doubt that a happy person enjoys the taste of life, and the level of his health is higher than that of an unhappy person. Happiness lowers the level of pressure and protects the heart. Research has shown that biological mechanism sexist that link happiness and joy to health. In order to arrive at happiness you have to work from the bottom upwards, from the body to the soul:

- To give the body the full right to enjoy health and immunity through exercise, correct diet and good sleep.
- To supply yourself with the existential needs of the soul and add movement, music and healing to your life, to leave the past, and to learn to live in and enjoy the present.
- To discover that you have everything you need to be happy, to enjoy what is there instead of suffering from what is not there.
- To arrive at a balance between common sense and emotion by giving expression to the heart and cognitive awareness
- To free yourself from the emotional scarring of the past without hesitating to receive help externally from efficacious systems
- To listen to the needs of the heart and not just to common sense – not being afraid of making big changes to the paths you have trodden till now that have just caused suffering
- To connect through meditation and contemplation with the source of the positive energy that allows you to implement your spiritual aspirations
- To strengthen your relationships with others who are the main source of satisfaction and enjoyment, to value and love yourself so that you can do this with others

- To learn to listen to your intuition, to give importance to the messages you receive in dreams, to take steps to increase your self confidence
- To work at realizing your aspirations and dreams in life

If we can work throughout this from a position of full awareness that life is temporary and that it serves us in our progress towards its source, then it will lead us to happiness, calm and freedom.

Dr Roger Walsh has done research and found eight important criteria that help sustain happiness, and mental and physical health [31]:

- Physical exercise: Aerobic exercise or weight training for at least 30 minutes.
- Proper diet and nutrition: it is important to keep to a healthy diet and especially to pay attention to Omega-3 which contains anti-inflammatory fatty acids in addition to many other health benefits (supplements are not enough – you have to consume fish from the North Sea, such as salmon); Vitamin D through controlled exposure to sunlight. There is a lack of this in most of the population, and it is important in the treatment and prevention of a great number of diseases.
- Time outdoors: Research has found that activities in natural surroundings improve your state of mind and contribute to health.
- Relationships: Conducting supportive relationships with the people close to us, helps us through difficulties and to live longer.
- Stress management and relief of tension: It has been found that activities such as meditation and yoga can relieve tension.
- Vacation: It is with rest for the body and mind that we maintain our health.

---

[31] www.drrogerwalsh.com/topics/lifestyle-and-mental-health

- Belief and spirituality: Research that has been conducted over many years has found that religious people who for years pray regularly, live longer lives.
- Service and contributing to others: It has been found that altruism and assistance to others help maintain body and soul, and that whoever has had an extreme experience, will be a better therapist, and this will also make a contribution to his own life.

Health imbalances

Signs of imbalances in health: Excess tension and lack of energy, nervousness, restlessness, over-emotionality, paleness. Depression and general discomfort can lead to a state of excess tension or a lack of energy. Every person who is charged with energy provides life and vitality to his tissues. This energy changes from day to day, with its amount and quality being influenced by both internal and external factors.

The internal factors depend on state of mind and on mental crises that cause blockages in energy. These blockages create an increase in stress, and as a result of this, stress also in the tissues and in various organs that is expressed in cramps, pain, ulcers in the small and large intestines and even in the brain (multiple sclerosis). The strength of the cramps affects state of mind and makes the person nervous, impatient, and unloved. This state of mind in turn affects the body and makes the first symptoms worse. In this way a vicious circle is established that only makes the problem worse and turns it into a chronic one.

External factors may exacerbate or alleviate the situation. Thus, for example, a person who has entered into a depression as a result of losing someone dear to him, eats food devoid of vitality, and does not sleep well, will just experience a deterioration in his condition.

On the other hand, a person who is in a state of depression, but consumes nutritious food such as fruit and vegetable juices, sleeps for sufficient hours (usually more than the normal), and does not waste energy, will experience an improvement in energy. As a result his state of depression will be short, and he will return to normal functioning.

A balanced person

The characteristics of a healthy person with a good level of vitality who does not suffer from excess stress:

- An upright body, a flexible spine, loose and strong muscles without difficultly in contracting or relaxing
- A facial expression full of life, with an easy smile, with no contractions between the eyes, and bright eyes
- Full, deep and slow breathing, with a brief pause after the breath, and uniform breathing rhythm
- Calm heartbeat, calm and regular pulse, normal blood pressure
- A soft belly, regular bowel movements, semi-solid stools with volume, light expulsion of gas without an odor of decomposition
- Among women: regular monthly periods with a lively red color to the discharge

Excess stress

The characteristics of an introverted person who doesn't know how to express his emotions and does not release his spiritual tension:

- The body seems bent and contracted either entirely or in certain areas
- The skin is pale and hard, and produces cold sweat
- The look in the eyes is tense, the expression hard and frozen, the forehead contracted, the lips pursed, the mouth is angled downwards as in an expression of sadness, there are creases around the lips, the eyes lack sparkle
- Tension in the muscles of the jaw, the throat, the chest and the spine, back pain, dryness in the mouth with a feeling of thirst during meals
- Shallow breathing accompanied by an interruption between breaths, a permanent feeling of heaviness and tightness in the chest without letup after a breath
- The heart is rigid and contracted, the pulse is fast, sharp and short, sometimes the pulse is irregular, high blood pressure
- Hard and contracted stomach, excess acidity in the stomach, indigestion, stomach ulcers, constipation or diarrhea, hemorrhoids
- Among women: irregular menstrual cycle with a small amount of blood
- Among men: a tough state of mind, an immediate nervous or angry response to minor external irritations, impatience, restlessness, difficulty in falling asleep, disturbances in sleep and early awakening

Stress in children

There is no doubt that tense parents raise nervous children. We have to remember that our young children, mainly up to kindergarten age, have not yet succeeded in developing methods of calming themselves and maintaining a state of mental and physical balance. This period is therefore critical for them and at home we should never create behavioral imprinting that is based on excess stress.

A good state of mind in the parents, even at times of stress, inspires a feeling of calmness and security in the child and imparts the ability to develop tools for dealing with similar situations in the future. Stressed parents project their distress onto their children, who absorb the stress and become pressured and worried in the face of any mission, small and large, that is placed before them.

Mental stress has a direct influence on the state of health of the children. It weakens the immune system, exposes the children to disease and causes headaches and stomach pain. Our role as parents is to identify signs that indicate a high level of stress in our young children.

Treatment for excess stress

- Regular physical activity that will promote deep breathing and increased perspiration
- Hot showers or swimming
- Emotional expression – to allow especially children to express their anger and to cry without inhibition
- Relaxation exercise such as meditation, bio-feedback and yoga

Level of vitality

Our bodies are charged with life energy influenced by many internal and external factors. The higher the life energy the more disease can be prevented and life extended.

Level of vitality and sunlight

We know intuitively that the body is more active and full of vitality when it is exposed to the sun. We therefore feel better in spring and summer. It is thus very important to listen to our bodies to evaluate its need to be exposed to the sun.

The importance of regulated and controlled exposure to sunlight:

- Improves toleration of personal stress and mental state
- Lowers the level of cholesterol in the blood
- Improves the efficiency of the immune system
- Increases physical ability and fitness to undertake physical effort
- Causes the production of vital hormones, and vitamin D, essential for the absorption of calcium and minerals
- Recharges the body with energy after illness or demanding work
- Prevents the development of infectious diseases and the multiplication of bacteria
- Reduces sleep disturbances and regulates the biological clock

Therefore it is desirable to be exposed to sunlight in every season in a controlled way that suits the individual without going as far as getting symptoms such as redness, itchiness, sunburn and pain as a consequence of over-exposure to the sun. You should be exposed to the sun only gradually and not for extended periods. You should take your children out to play in the open air.

Lack of energy

A state of lack of energy is created because of the continuing loss of emotional energy as a result of long-term mental crises, continued internal conflict, eating of food lacking in vitality, excessive physical work, minimum sleep, and loneliness without support or external help.

From the mental point of view a lack of energy is expressed by depression, the need to sleep, difficulty in getting up in the morning, and a lack of will to function. Among children the symptoms will be restlessness, lack of concentration and hyperactivity, fear and states of anxiety.

Treatment for lack of energy:

- Avoid aggressive activity
- Avoid loneliness and crying
- Avoid extended showers or baths and swimming in a pool
- Avoid drinking alcohol
- Reduce time spent sitting in front of a computer
- Increase drinking of fresh fruit and vegetable juices (with care when the inflammation is active)
- Avoid eating processed foods
- Sleep for more hours at night

The presence of loved ones, support and love, is the most important way of dealing with children and people with a low level of vitality.

The large intestine

The large intestine comprises the last stage in the digestive system in which the liquid of the food residue is absorbed and the contents turn from liquid to solids. Behind the proper functioning of the large intestine there are various physiological processes, among them the absorption of liquids and salts, rhythmic contractions and relaxations that mix the contents and conduct the feces to the rectum.

The emotional view: Excess stress that is connected to fear in the face of criticism (in a symbolic way the fear of criticism resembles the fear of expelling gas) and the fear of the possibility of physical injury, cause an increase in the level of stress in the abdominal cavity, mainly in the large intestine, which can be expressed in the appearance of ulcers in the mucosa of the intestine and in chronic inflammation in the bowel. In less severe cases diarrhea will occur.

Fear of criticism causes a person to keep his feelings in his stomach and not to share them, something that causes a lack of balance in the functioning of the large intestine. As time goes by the basic level of stress in the intestine increases until a physical disease appears. Incorrect eating habits catalyze the damage to proper functioning, while acceptable physical activity and the drinking of liquids between meals assist in reducing stress in the intestine and in balancing its functioning. It is therefore highly recommended that you encourage children to express their feelings and to emphasize their positive sides in place of continual criticism of negative things.

The small intestine

The small intestine begins at the exit from the stomach and ends at the large intestine, and forms the main part of the digestive system. It is a winding tube of seven to nine meters in length, with a diameter of about three centimeters, and it fills most of the space in the abdomen. The small intestine is divided into three parts: the duodenum, the jejunum and the ileum.

The small intestine has two main functions:

- The chemical digestion of food – carbohydrates, proteins and fats – into single sugars, amino acids, glycerol and into fatty acids respectively
- The absorption of minerals for the blood

The contraction mechanism exists thanks to the local nervous system which is affected and controlled by the central nervous system, which in turn is directly affected by mental state and daily stress.

Dysfunction in the small intestine leads to a change in the absorption process, which is manifested in weight loss, inflammation in the mouth and swelling in the intestines as a result of gas and diarrhea. Many people who suffer from absorption problems suffer also from a lack of blood as a result of the defective functioning in the absorption of iron, vitamin B12 or folic acid. They also tend to suffer from bone pain and muscle cramps as a result of a lessened absorption of calcium, and from a lowering in the absorption of vitamin K.

The mental view: A mental problem that causes a disturbance in the functioning of the small intestine stems from the difficulty in taking advantage of opportunities at the right time and to derive benefit from them. The suffering is connected with the feeling of having missed a chance of improving quality of life, difficulties in taking meaningful decisions, and difficulties in distinguishing right from wrong, good from bad, and feelings of guilt. All these cause stress and bring about cramps.

Meditation

Meditation is a system that assists in healing the body and quieting consciousness. In a state of meditation, through full self-awareness, we completely disregard the temptations that surround us. In this way we can connect with what we believe in, strengthen the soul in the deepest layers of consciousness that cause a person to change his relationship with himself and with the world around him. It's a simple easy technique that does not require effort but if you want it to succeed you will need discipline and persistence.

There are several meditation systems. What is common to all of them is that it is important to devote an hour regularly to sitting in a quiet place. It is possible to light a candle or listen to calming music. It is possible either to meditate standing up, or to sit on a chair with your back straight, your head and neck relaxed, your feet on the floor and your hands resting on your knees. It is possible to sit on the floor in the "lotus" position or to squat with your back straight, your head and neck relaxed and your hands resting on your knees.

Research proves that meditation strengthens the immune system and in a significant way diminishes unhealthy emotional states such as worry, depression, tiredness and confusion, and significantly raises the level of vitality. Research has shown that meditation reduces the rate of visits to the doctor by 50%, as it does with hospital admissions and the chances of heart disease and cancer and thus improves the mental state and cognitive ability. In addition to this, meditation extends life by about 22%, improves health, short- and long-term memory, and creates happiness.

Music

The capacity of music to heal the soul is known in all cultures. From the moment we are born, music accompanies us in both happy and sad times. An entire field of music therapy exists. Research has revealed that music lowers blood pressure and reduces pain and stress. The combination of music with guided imagery, or even music alone can serve as an alternative method to healing or meditation. There is appropriate music for every state of health and age group, and the rhythm needs to be individually matched.

Examples from various reports around the world of the positive effect of music:

- **For stress**: Roderigo's Concerto d'Aranjuez, Vivaldi's Four Seasons, Mozart's Symphony No 36
- **For stomach problems**: Handel's Concerto No 4, Vivaldi's Spring Concerto, Telemann's Mass
- **For low energy**: Sibelius' Karelia Suite, Rossini's William Tell Overture
- **For reinforcing hope and inner strength**: Schubert's Ave Maria, Beethoven's Ninth Symphony

A new way

After a number of years of relative quiet I did not feel well. It was in the spring of 2011. After a deterioration that continued for a few months, I was treated on and off with steroids and antibiotics in addition to Imuran, and still the CRP (C-reactive protein —C-reactive protein is an acute-phase protein which is a measurement of the level of inflammation) jumped at times to 20 and I often suffered from pain. Sometimes the stomach pains continued for many weeks. I could have up to seven bowels movements in a day, and my general feeling was really not good at all. The doctors had no answer to this beyond their recommendation to increase the drugs. I agreed to this because I felt I had no option.

At the same time I was the father of two children, and I was working at a start-up company that greatly interested me. The work, however, was hard and intensive. About two years had gone by since I had published the first edition of my book. I received many responses from people with Crohn's or Colitis or their relatives, who told me how much the book had helped them and had encouraged them to make a change in their lives to improve the state of their health. I was confident of the recommendations in my book – a calm lifestyle, monitoring and treatment, and diet – a result of my monitoring and self-study over the years, but I felt that I myself was not succeeding in fully implementing the recommendations, and as a result of that there were times when the state of my health was not how it should be. I had strictly maintained the monitoring and treatment, and I continued to undergo tests and visit the doctor regularly. When it came to diet, I did succeed in sticking to it and for more than seven years I did not eat out. This was perhaps relatively easy because the response of the body is immediate and clear when you eat badly. However, I did not succeed in fully maintaining a calm lifestyle that met the requirements of my body.

Many people asked me why I wrote the book. Beyond the sense of mission and the desire to help people in my condition, I also wanted to help myself. I wanted that the instructions that had proved themselves over years would not be forgotten and would remain clear. About six years had passed since I had the operation. After the operation I had promised myself to write down my conclusions concerning the disease so that I would not forget them, and so that I wouldn't return to a lifestyle that didn't suit my health. With time, however, I missed this goal. When you feel better you forget the hard times and you live life with all its intensity, and when the signs of the disease begin to return, there is denial. We say "It'll be alright". We continue with our lives as usual, and we forget to listen to our bodies. We say to ourselves: "What – now that I'm finally feeling good, I shouldn't take a bite of something that I really love, although I know that it could give me stomach pain?"

After consultations, it was recommended to me that I begin with Humira treatment – a biological medication based on human antibodies and which is given, in my case, by injection once a week or every two weeks. Like Imuran, Humira also depresses the immune system and both are meant to work together to suppress the inflammation in a better way and for longer.

After about a month of taking the medication, I felt a lot better, but still not excellent. The doctor recommended increasing the dose to one shot a week, and then my condition really improved. About two months after starting the treatment I could join in at the family meal, eat pita bread with a beef cutlet (which until two months before, I would have refused) and – nothing! Nothing! Not a twinge in my stomach. No noise, no stirring, no cramps, no pain, not even in the slightest, not even the awful feeling of the food passing through the various parts of the bowel. I remembered what it was like to be healthy, how it was not to feel your intestine after every meal.

I felt good. I kept to the correct diet, and although my condition was good, I wasn't tempted to eat rubbish. I continued with my intensive lifestyle at my work at the start-up and dealing with my two small and fantastic children. I continued taking the Imuran and Humira, and I felt generally good. The blood tests also confirmed this and the CRP measurement was close to zero.

However, after about six months the well-known sounds of war in my stomach area returned. There was a kind of unpleasant feeling and there were strange digestive sounds after I finished a meal. At first there was of course denial – it's just a virus, it will obviously pass. It is amazing, how after all the years that I had Crohn's, there was still denial. After about two weeks, I did not doubt, as I had done many times in the past, that the inflammation had returned. Blood tests showed that the CRP measurement had jumped to 11. That meant that there was active inflammation in my body, and there was no doubt that it was Crohn's disease.

It was very difficult feeling. I had Crohn's disease for sixteen years, treated with the most modern drugs that western medicine could offer and the inflammation continued to run wild in my bowel. I had no doubt that I was about to go through a very difficult time. It wasn't long before the pain returned to various parts of my stomach, especially in the area where I had the operation. I was flooded with memories from the time before the operation.

I was sent for an MRI test (there is nothing like drinking a little Barium to improve your state of mind). I got the results back after a few days. In the envelope there were two pages of medical analysis of the test results that described what was going on in my stomach. I didn't imagine that after the operation I still had so much left of my intestine. Why could I not, just for once, open the envelope and find a note that said "All is well"?

According to the results the inflammation had spread to nearly every the part of the small intestine and beyond it, and now also to the large intestine, and there was narrowing of inflamed areas with all the rest of the symptoms.

The long silence in the rooms of the Gastro doctor who had received the test results announced to me that the situation was not good.

My sharp instincts had taught me to identify these long silences as a bad sign.

The doctor recommended an immediate change in my medication treatment, which included various antibiotics and a return to the steroids. Worse than that, the conclusion was that there was no option other than another operation.

"You have narrowing. The pain you are feeling is because of the narrow parts of the intestine, and you therefore have to have an operation before it's too late."

"What does that mean – 'too late'?" I asked, even though I knew the answer.

"Before there is a blockage in the bowel and then you will need an emergency operation. In this kind of operation, they will open the entire abdomen, which is not like a planned operation in which you can choose the surgeon and it is possible to use a laparoscopy, which will not require a complete opening of the abdomen."

"And what will happen after the operation? Both us know that the disease won't go away."

To this she had no answer.

Just six years had passed since my first operation. I couldn't believe that within such a short space of time I would be back at the same point. The memories of the first operation were too fresh for me to run and have another. I could think of a thing or two that I would prefer to do more than waking up in surgery ward B connected to tubes from every orifice (also from orifices that were not there before).

There is no doubt that this was the crisis point.

I consulted five more Gastro experts, but I didn't receive the response I wanted from any of them. Some of them supported the approach that it was worth going for the operation, some said that there was no need to hurry because the disease wasn't going to go away, and that in my present state it was not advisable to operate because it would be hard for me to recover.

From the medication perspective all that I could opt for next was Remicaid, a drug that suppresses the immune system. It was not innovative like Humira, and was not based on human antibodies. Although I had heard from a few people about various sensitivities to Remicaid, I decided to implement the recommendation to stop the Humira treatment, and to change to Remicaid.

During that period the pain went on for weeks, so in addition to all these drugs, every two weeks there were antibiotics to help calm the situation. They did not contribute to balance in the body, however. Unlike Humira, treatment with Remicaid is done under supervision via infusion at hospital. Sitting for half a day in the gastro ward connected to an infusion did not improve my state of mind. It reminded me of days that I really wanted to forget. This session with Remicaid was short, however, because on top of all these troubles I got pneumonia, which together with my stomach pushed both my

CRP measurement and my pain sky-high. The winter of 2012 did not go by easily.

Further rounds of consultations with doctors who put forward various approaches concerning subsequent treatment and the progress towards the operation, only clarified for me that they really didn't know what to do with a patient like me. The situation was dispiriting, and out of this despair I took a step that I had not taken since my operation. I completely stopped all the medication and took a break from the doctors. I just wanted to rest, both physically and mentally.

During that period, just as the period after the operation, I was lying at home more, and I had time to think about what had brought me to this state. I had lived my life according to the recommendations of my own book, and according to what I had recommended to many other patients who like me, were looking for solutions to a disease that is not clear, I had maintained a diet that I thought was right for me, and for many years I had taken care not to eat out. Under continual monitoring, I had made sure to do all the tests, and I visited the doctors at least once every few months. And still my medical condition did not stabilize.

However, on closer examination, I understood that I was not really keeping to the all the components of the lifestyle-monitoring-nutrition pyramid. My lifestyle at that time was not calm. I was working at the start-up where the work was interesting but very stressful, and included long hours. I often had to travel for about an hour every morning and evening, and in addition, my two wonderful children, aged four and two required a lot of attention like all children their age. It was impossible to call this a calm lifestyle. The state of my health did not allow me to have a normal family life and to work in the way they expected of me there.

It's hard to make a change, and even harder to make a change when you are not feeling well. You feel a lack of confidence. What kind of confidence can someone whose stomach hurts from morning to night have – a person who goes to the bathroom at least five times a day? However, I decided that my life was not going in a good direction and that it was up to me to do everything I could to make a change.

Because I had a family to support, I couldn't simply resign from work. I decided to look for work at a distance of no more than twenty minutes' drive from the house, and no less importantly, a job that would include a calm work environment, with nice people and normal hours. I decided that when I went into job interviews I would leave the disease outside. It didn't matter how much it was hurting me, I would not let it affect my conduct. And if I would be asked about it, I would use just a dry description to explain the disease from which I suffered.

Despite the state of my health, it did not take long for me to find a suitable place, close to home and very calm, and after a month I already couldn't imagine working in any other way.

My health situation might not have improved in the new workplace, but it didn't significantly deteriorate either. I was able to cope better with the situation because my new lifestyle suited the state of my health better, although I knew that without the medication my condition could deteriorate at any time, because as I had already learned, it could always be worse (but it also could always be better).

At the same time, the hand of fate led me to a meeting with Adi Zusman, nutritionist and health coach. She said that she had read my book, and that she had wanted to meet me. During the times when I don't feel well, I'm really not enthusiastic with people about my disease, or about starting new treatments. However, because I had not come across the concept of "health coach", and certainly not a coach for Crohn's patients, out of politeness and curiosity I agreed to meet with her. During a conversation of about an hour Adi explained to me that health coaching helps patients to cope with their disease and guides them on how to take decisions regarding their lifestyle and health. As she spoke I felt that there was definitely a place for guidance like this. Many patients are confused and in desperate need of knowledge that will help them deal better with the disease. This was the reason that I had written the book, but my stomach pains were not strengthening my patience. Suddenly I saw in front of my eyes all those therapists who understood absolutely nothing about my disease and had pretended to sell me drugs that were discovered to be useless at best, and at worst, harmful. I asked her: "Does it really help? Is it possible to point to one patient who suffered from this disease and who was really helped by health coaching?"

And then Adi told me about Eran Roter, a Crohn's patient who suffered greatly from the disease, and who was today living in a healthy way and managed to take part in iron man competitions which demand a level of physical fitness that would challenge even healthy people. Eran studied and became a health coach himself.

I knew quite a few Crohn's and Colitis patients, people in whom the disease breaks out only seldom, and patients who suffer regularly from the disease and who are forced to live with an active illness, very often with the help of drugs. It is rare to come across a patient who has been in a serious condition and who has succeeded in returning to a normal lifestyle, and what's more, has participated in challenging sporting competitions.

I decided to meet with Eran and to see with my own eyes if this was really the case. At the meeting we exchanged more than a few experiences. Eran told me about various admissions to hospital that he had and about his difficult times with the disease, which very much reminded me of what I had experienced at exactly the same time. He said that his nutrition was based on a diet called "The Specific Carbohydrate Diet". He offered me to train with him. The training included ten personal meetings in which I would learn how to analyze various situations in my life. In this way I would be able to identify sources of stress in my life and to cope with various situations that are created by Crohn's disease.

Because I had gone through more than a few strange and varied treatments and the cost of this training was not negligible, I was very skeptical. If after all I had experienced and learned during the sixteen years of my disease, did I now need someone to teach me how to manage my life? On the other hand I had to be honest with myself and to admit that despite everything I knew and did, the state of my health was not good. Eventually, after much hesitation, I decided to try and do the health coaching with Eran and to begin with the Specific Carbohydrate Diet.

At that time my diet had been based on white bread morning and night, pasta and rice at lunchtime and lots of sugar for energy – things that are forbidden in the Specific Carbohydrate Diet. Because I didn't feel good, I had also not been eating vegetables and fruit, meat and many other things that I knew made me feel unwell. If I had to do without bread and rice, what would be left for me to eat? I knew that the worst thing was to be hungry, because in a state of hunger it is hard to make the correct decisions concerning diet.

☐

During the first two months I stopped eating bread, and I began eating more eggs (hard-boiled, not fried). Later I added more cooked chicken with vegetables in a soup. I gradually reduced both the rice and the pasta. I substituted the sugar with lots of honey. At the beginning I was eating a great deal of chicken. Afterwards I discovered that fish is easier to digest, and I began eating a fish a day, simply cooked in the oven with cooked vegetables – mainly zucchini and carrot. As my condition improved a little I discovered that I could eat bananas (even if it was in small amounts) which revealed themselves as an excellent source of energy, and greatly helped to stop the diarrhea. After a few weeks I began eating two bananas a day with natural goat's milk yoghurt and honey. Between meals I drank herbal tea with honey, and I always had dates on me, and later also nuts which kept me from reaching a state of hunger, and maintained the level of energy in my body.

In addition to the health exercises and the diet change, I decided, after a break of a few months, to go back to taking Imuran and Humira. Because I wanted to be certain that I was doing everything to improve the state of my health, I decided in addition to get the help of medicinal cannabis in the form of powder and drops, that helped ease the pain and improve the quality of my sleep, which is so important for the body in the recovery from the inflammation.

During the course of the exercises with Eran I learned to contemplate my daily life and to identify various situation of stress. Later I learned how I could neutralize these situations or how not to arrive at them at all. I am sure that, as in every area, in health coaching there are better coaches than others, and a particular coach may not necessarily suit everyone, although this is an additional tool that can help you improve your condition. One of the most important things I learned from the coaching was to free some time during the week for exercises that would calm me. This mission always seemed very hard at the beginning, especially as there were small children in the house, but was definitely possible. For me there is only one place to do this, and that's the sea. I began swimming in the sea at least once a week, and my wife supported me in this. I discovered that this exercise served me as a source of energy for the whole week. Not only ill people, but everyone should set aside a regular time for exercise that will do them good and cleanse them of their everyday difficulties. I know patients who swim in a pool, and others who claim that yoga does them good. Everyone can find that one thing which is like breathing pure oxygen, like pressing restart on a computer – an exercise that once you've done it you feel better and can cope better with the disease and the challenges it places before you. Don't stop seeking till you find the physical exercise that does you good. When you find the right activity you will know it.

About two months after starting the diet and the coaching, I felt an improvement. There was less pain and diarrhea. After about four months the situation improved even more. This showed also in the blood tests when the CRP inflammation measurement began to go down. After about six months I began to put on weight, even though I had completely stopped carbohydrates and sugar. For the first time in years I did not have an active inflammation in my body for a period of months. My CRP count went down to zero. In consultation with the doctor I began to reduce the medication. Nine months after I had started the diet and the coaching (which lasted about two months) I put on 5kg – from 57kg at the time when I had not been feeling well, I went up to 62kg. My CRP continued to stay at zero, even though I had reduced the drug dosage.

I feel much better and confident in my health and its stability. I still have days when I don't feel well, and sometimes there is a little pain, but my recovery from it is a lot faster that it had been in the past. I continue to be under medical monitoring, and in the not-so-good times I continue to get help from medication. I remember to give my body the rest it needs and I continue to record and strictly monitor my diet, my weight and the state of my health, so that it will be easier for me to identify what's working and what's not.

It may well be that health coaching and the SCD Diet don't suit every patient. I'm not sure that at every stage of my disease I would have been prepared to experiment with these treatments, but they helped me to get through a difficult time when the inflammation broke out. These are additional tools in the toolbox of Crohn's and Colitis patients for coping with the disease.

My new way is in fact a process in which I discovered again what works for me in this period of my life and condition of the disease. From this period I learned once again of the body's wonderful ability to recover from difficult situations despite the opinions of various doctors. It is important to remember this, especially when there is pain and despair takes over, and it seems as if nothing that can be done. There is always something that can be done, and there is always something to learn. Even after sixteen years of active inflammation, and countless attempts, I learned something new about myself. I am certain, that like me, any patient can make a change in his lifestyle and his diet that will improve the state of his health.

"A journey of a thousand miles begins with a single step"
– Lao Tzu

Your first step is to want to feel better.

From hospital bed to coaching

This chapter is written by Eran Roter, health coach and Crohn's patient.

The royal way

When you can't move from the bed because you are in pain, you're nauseous and every movement you make raises anxiety and pain in various parts of your body – only one thing remains: you. You are there alone with your fears and pain, questioning yourself about existence and the meaning of life, when you discover the simple truth. And that truth is the present.

Without regrets about the past, without fears for the future, the present introduces you to the person most dear to you in the entire universe: you yourself. And in this meeting, there are only winners, because if I don't love myself in the mirror, I can talk to myself and understand where the thoughts come from that have led to a feeling so bad – to understand that it is feelings and thoughts like these that stand between what I am now and what I want to be. It's not what I want to receive, nor what I want to achieve, but what I want to be.

Just presence in the present: paying full attention to what is happening now allows me to live with even the most difficult feeling that might appear, and to let it pass as a storm does. And after the storm, comes the clean-up – like a mountain road after the rain has washed away all the accumulated oil and dust. And when the sun bursts out between the clouds and shines its first beams, you can dry the tears in your eyes, and look down with pride. To celebrate the present and to see the path that I choose, based on what I love and what I want more than anything else.

When I was in hospital and during all the months that I was in bed at home, it was not the disease that prostrated me – it was my diminished life and my lack of ability to see the present that struck me clearly. I rediscovered the meaning of this, when I met myself again and I realized again just how much I liked myself, and when I was able to thank God for the life He had given me. Despite the difficulties I experienced at that time, I discovered a few things that worked to my benefit. I discovered the hand that was stretched out to me, that I hadn't been aware of. Actually, I had been aware of attempts to help, only I hadn't accepted them, because I had been busy with an internal war which prevented me from seeing where I was stepping. The meaning of choice in life means that I don't need pain to remind me that I am alive, and pain is not necessary for learning. The meaning of choice in life means living in the moment in calmness and to rely on yourself if life brings you a new mystery that you have not learned how to solve, that you'll be able to ask the right questions, and to be helped by the right people so that you can progress in the search for the right questions that will bring you in time to an answer or answers that you cannot imagine at the moment, but that when they come, will seem obvious.

It's not possible without this process. Einstein said that on the way to a single great success you sometimes make a thousand mistakes. You have to learn to accept as part of the process of learning, to pick yourself up every time, and continue. He also said that asking the right questions is the way to creative thought, discovery and invention. Einstein's genius lay not just in his thought and his brilliant theories, but in his presentation of the right questions that led to new insights.

Paying attention – a small thing that makes a big difference

Seven years ago the picture looked different. My health was not in my control and my feeling was that my entire life was deteriorating and was slipping through my fingers. Every time I tried to take hold of something stronger, every time that I made an effort to do something that would work in returning control to me, it escaped from my hands and I was vanquished. Nothing that I had known up to that time worked. I tried everything that I thought would work and the situation just became more and more depressing, until I reached complete hopelessness. There, at the age of thirty-five, I met myself again. During my third admission to hospital I understood that the problem was not that what I was doing was not working, but rather it was the way I was doing it and the way I was experiencing the reality I was trying to change.

My son Yuval, built a tower out of Lego. He showed it to me to show off with something impressive. When I looked with appreciation at the tower he had built, I was reminded of myself as a child, enjoying building with Lego and each time creating something from those wonderful blocks. The tower was built out of lots of blocks and different colors – red, yellow, black, white, green and more, straight blocks, corner blocks, and blocks for the roof. My health was built in the same way out of various parts, various areas of life. When I looked at the tower standing on the table, it seemed obvious that it was there and that I was accepting it as it existed and that I could continue onwards. It is the details of the tower, however, like those of our health, that make it whole. Without the red or black blocks, the tower would not have stood, or it would have been lower. In the same way one can view a diet that was good for me, or the time that I dedicate to myself, the breaks, time for planning and more. These are important details. Their result is good health, and today I know I need to pay attention to them, and allocate them a part in my daily reality.

Every single area of my life that is important to me, and whose effect I am aware of, can be manifested in emotion and health. The possibility of listening to the body's signals and what they express, of paying attention to details, and the capability of making a difference – that's what I want to get across here.

Between self-discipline and self-listening

Self-discipline emanates from meaning. Discipline must come from a place of something meaningful to me, because then it is real to me, and "holds water" for an extended time.

These days it's easy for me to listen to myself because I can, more quickly, read the signs that my body transmits. For example, I ate chicken for lunch, and I planned to eat salad and perhaps another side dish with it. I was quite hungry before the meal, but I felt satisfied after the first chicken thighs that I ate. My stomach began to turn a little inside and raised the question: Should I eat more, and how much?

As I listen to my children telling me during the meal about their day, I make place in my thoughts and feelings also for my stomach and for every other part of my body that speaks to me, so that I can decide how to continue with the meal. Because I ate a full breakfast in the morning, and a snack with vegetables, I decided to give up on the side dishes in this meal. I can eat salad afterwards. This entire internal debate took a few minutes, and didn't occupy me beyond that. The feeling is one of satiety and tiredness, and on a hot day with a few hours of work still to come, even before this listening to my body, it is important to listen to the request to forego another portion and to give myself an extra break before the rest of the day's activities.

Listening to yourself is exactly this.

Simple?

Yes it is – after getting used to it, and after self-listening training, and out of an awareness of the price I will pay if I don't listen to the body's signals. It's clear to me and to whoever deals with this field, that this process of listening and remembering to listen to ourselves is not always simple. And that's the reason why I chose coaching as a way of helping. What comes out of the process isn't always easy, but it is always fascinating and always teaches something. Broadly speaking, what I say is: Everyone can.

In order to illustrate the moments in which I understood that I really wasn't attentive and not listening to what my body was transmitting to me, I'm going to take you back seven years, to the lowest and most painful period of my life. I was a successful deputy marketing manager who, out of a search for a professional challenge and a new business field, had become a business consultant.

After being admitted three times to hospital I was diagnosed in 2005 as a Crohn's patient. Four months after the diagnosis I was admitted for the fourth time with a systemic collapse after I had taken a blow from life.

It began when, for a change, the combined medicinal treatment I was receiving began working, and over three weeks I began to feel an easing of my pains and a reduction in my amount of daily bowel movements. I did what I knew how to do, or thought would work on the basis of my past experience, and I returned to running a little to improve my low state of mind, and to try and bounce my health back to what it had been.

Within a very short space of time I was training for a run of 10km and I was registered for a professional race. As the race neared I was not feeling good, and I performed exercises with myself to try and concentrate on the goal I had set for myself. After about 2.5 km and the first hill of the race, I felt I had hit the wall, and I stopped running. I finished the race at a walk. I sat down behind the finish line, and that was it. It was not easy to move beyond that point. I was evacuated to the emergency medical center, and then straight to hospital. In retrospect I understood that it was only because of my intense will that I managed to finish the race at a walk.

It turned out that I had pneumonia and a flare-up of Crohn's at the same time. As a result of this, and in addition, I had been dehydrated, and had required a few infusions to get back on my feet.

I woke up early the following morning. I was in hospital, cut off from home and my daily worries, quietly preparing a tasty cup of tea and looking at the view of the city from the western window, breathing in the air of the city coming to life and awakening to the new day before it.

I feel that just as I am able to enjoy as if for the first time the cup of tea I had prepared for myself, and these few moments of perspective in the morning, I want it to be like this all my life. Then I understand that I have reached the bottom, because I turn around and face the internal medicine ward again, breathe deeply and realize that it isn't working. It isn't working – not because of what I'm doing, because it's clear that there is something to learn – but because of the way I see, feel, smell, breathe, taste and listen to reality. The thoughts I amused to thinking on any particular subject affect emotion, and vice versa. I understand that if I could learn about myself again from the beginning through a slightly different way of seeing reality, I would be able to discover new things that might perhaps work, and perhaps the path that would open before me would be easier than the one I had experienced until now. I didn't have any answers, just a new way of seeing the questions, and the belief that I could.

I learned later that this was a process of "paradigm shift", or "change of perception", and I learned the importance of belief and how to be helped by it and to help with it.

The story ends two days after my admission. A good friend comes to fetch me from the hospital, and takes me home. I feel something different in the air and wonder how my children and wife will accept someone who has barely functioned for a few months. When I enter the house the children jump on me with happiness. I sit at the table and they settle on me, hugging me strongly. Tears of excitement stream from my eyes, a good feeling of fatherhood that completes the new path that I have begun.

I take a deep breath and continue on the journey whose fruits I enjoy every day, but whose hardships I don't wish on anyone.

Learning all over again to rely on yourself

How do you get back to relying on yourself when everything is hurting in your body and all your systems are failing? I had taken the first step and put belief back in my life. With the belief came a new understanding. Everything that had been said in the past few months, by the doctors, dieticians and Crohn's patients that I had met – everything they had advised, suddenly sounded to me so incorrect. As long as I had been fighting and had been so vague and distracted with the fear and anger that had accompanied every experience, I had not really listened. I had not been open to accepting the help that had been offered to me, because I had been so busy with my internal struggle and the struggle with the disease. But the minute that I accepted the situation and I stopped asking "Why did this have to happen to me?" I understood that to enjoy the cup of tea in the morning, to give myself a few minutes of perspective – that was the main, and not the unimportant, thing. Through these moments that I devote to myself, I direct awareness to the here and now and dismantle the barriers in favor of a new clarity. The wonderful thing is that still today, after years of feeling good without medication, these moments are more precious to me than any other thing during the day, because through them I am free to feel my body, and I give myself time to bring the tempo of my thoughts down almost to a stop.

This stoppage or these pauses that I devote to myself allow me to speak to myself on a deeper and clearer level. There I meet everything that I have inside and allow it to rise. Whether it's fear or anger that has accumulated, I meet it, and learn to understand it. If it's pain or discomfort in my stomach I breathe into the pain, and allow it to exist. In this way I have learned to live with myself in peace. Being at one with every emotion, whether it's a difficult or easy one, allows my body to tell me what is not good for me. It creates space in my thoughts for doing the right thing for myself in order to return to the feeling that things are good for me. The meaning of learning all over again to rely on yourself is to understand that there are things that you can learn today: about yourself, about the world, about your health. And then, out of awareness, you ask the right questions.

To trust yourself means knowing that what you do not know is within reach, and all that you need to do is to admit that you do not know to investigate the question that is bothering you.

"Mankind need not fear the unknown if it is capable of achieving what it needs and it wants." Paulo Coelho, The Alchemist.

In this way I set out every morning on a journey on which I discovered anew what is good for me, and what does not contribute to my health. I collected information from all my meetings with the dieticians and I began to actualize the advice that I received and that I knew worked. I listened more to the people I met who were living a full life with Crohn's. I listened to the therapists who help people to rise above bad thoughts and to try a new diet that works for them. Every morning I began with a tasty cup of tea that I prepared for myself, and a few moments of quiet and listening to myself and to my body. Every morning I reminded myself of the belief I came to face within the confines of the hospital, and of the decision that I am open to learning new things about myself that work to the good of my health.

I received help from my wife who encouraged me to go out for walks in the mornings when it was physically hard for me to get of bed, and insisted that I would learn to cook the new dishes that I had discovered were healthy for me. She was not prepared to accept me as a patient who was dependent on her and I responded positively to the challenge, fueled myself with belief every time that I felt bad. From day to day I got used to drawing strength from my belief and to give up on thoughts that lead to difficult emotions. At the same time the change in diet that I had begun to implement for myself began to show positive signs. Three weeks after I had moved to a liquids-only diet, for the first time in years the diarrhea stopped, and the pains came down to a tolerable level. The more that the pain was reduced, the more I was able to enthusiastically occupy myself with my research on myself on the subject of diet. I knew that I could not continue to live on liquids alone for an extended time and I therefore continued to read and to get advice, and each time to implement something new that I thought would work. During this period I already knew that I was learning to eat all over again, absolutely like a baby, but I waited with experimenting with a new type of solid food that friends with Crohn's had told me about. In 2007, after I had read the book by Eileen Rothschild on the Specific Carbohydrate Diet (SCD) and internalized the rationale behind it, I began with this diet when I felt confident in my path. I continued to implement the things that I had learned about myself in the preceding weeks, while I completely gave up bread and starchy foods for the sake of my new health.

To trust yourself is to know that in the moment of crisis you may not have the right answer, but you will certainly know how to ask the right question that will lead you to learning and finding a solution that will work. Today I know that prior to starting SCD, there was a preparation period of a few weeks of introspection and learning that helped with the change. The approach was to try something new every day or two, or to restore to the stomach something you would never have dared to before. Thus alongside of the SCD rationale that I believe in to this day, I built a new diet for myself with an abundance of tasty foods. As the weeks and months went by I returned to enjoying food, and to preparing fuller and more filling meals. I learned that snacks between meals ease the stomach and also help me to maintain high energy. I found that there were foods that were not good for me in the morning, but were fine if I ate them at lunch or in the evening.

The connection with intuition, and the feeling that I could trust myself, persisted. As time went by and I notched up successes, I was able to listen more to what my body, and not just my stomach, was saying to me during meals. When I felt less good, I was more easily able to answer the question: was it something I ate, was it the need to rest, was it stress, a particular emotion? The fog lifted and dissipated. After five months I registered for a personal training course with the aim to return to fulltime work.

On limiting belief and parallel belief

When I returned home after my fourth admission to hospital, I understood that I could live differently. I didn't know exactly what I would do, or how I would do it, but I began to change the limiting belief that I had at the time. The belief that limited my field of vision was that I alone knew what was good for me, and that I alone would decide what I would eat or what I would do. In the framework of this belief, which can also be positive, there was a delaying belief according to which I was acting. And that was that when I wasn't feeling good, my way of comforting myself was to eat something that I liked although I knew it would harm me. The compensation would only bring more pain and that pain would distance me from the ability to broaden my awareness so that I could accept new things in my world. In this way I was left stranded in a cycle of suffering. When I understood that the quiet that I devoted to myself – and the emphasis is on "devote to myself" and not on waiting for someone to offer it to me on a silver tray – that quiet allows me to experience life with perspective and to approach more difficult challenges with balance and direction. I trained myself to give time to myself, to accept perspective and to allow all the difficult emotions to surface. What remained was clear and pleasant thought.

It took me a few months to arrive at this change in belief, which I call "parallel belief". With parallel belief there are many challenges in different directions because you are aware of pain, anger, the sense of guilt and the frustration that flows from parallel/limiting belief, and I don't always know what to do to avoid them. On the other hand you can see that in situations in which your behavior is a little different, the results are to your benefit.

This is the place to note the amazing feeling of the celebration of victory. When did you last celebrate the fact that you felt good for a week, a month, three months, even a day? Think of the value of the victory celebration as an incentive that provides inspiration to continue the process and try to celebrate the milestone as a step on the path to health and not just the finish line.

I know that if I go back to behaving as I once did, or more correctly, to have my behavior managed for me, I increase the chances of an outbreak of Crohn's. I thus developed an awareness and a higher sensitivity to the signs that my body sends me and I adopted many more personal tools that I use every time that I feel a small deterioration in the state of my health.

The small details

If I've learned that a break of five to ten minutes in the morning can help me to concentrate and to play my part to the fullest, why give it up? And if I know that eating carbohydrates with fried food when my stomach is not quiet can cause an even bigger mess, why should I take the chance?

These are small, important details that I learned out of introspection and the understanding that I had once thought that I could avoid getting through the day without a break or without giving up on tempting food. However, when I look at the wider picture I can see just how these small details have a big effect on health.

When I give myself a break, I allow my head and body to rest from the continuous activity, and when I return to activity I'm more alert and effective at work. When I eat correctly, I know when it's alright to eat a heavy meal and when I should eat a light meal. My approach is that we should begin the change where it's easy for us and not in where it's hard for us to make a change. This is the reason that as a coach I let the person I'm coaching look at and observe himself and learn about his behavior before he begins to change things. Our awareness has amazing power. The more we give it more space and pay attention to the small details that affect our daily balance, the better we can know what affects our physical feelings more and what affects them less.

The preparation and the planning for change are very important. However, the beginning has to be easy and not difficult, so that we can deal with the change over time. If it's easy for you to begin with something big, go for it. However, if big change frightens or daunts you, it's normal. That's why most people don't make changes easily. The best way is to look for the small things that affect your feelings of confidence and increase your feelings of capability. If the change is in the field of sport and you begin with fitness exercises once a week, enjoy it because it's the correct step and your body will already begin to feel every small change that occurs. Remember that the tallest building in New York is built out of strong beams and bolts, good glass, concrete, insulation and more. Every detail in that building is as important as every component of your health.

Once I had adjusted to the knowledge I had gained from the Specific Carbohydrate Diet (SCD) I moved from the liquid diet to a very solid diet that I got from the nutritionist. At this stage I recognized the benefits of the change of diet and learned to appreciate every small step I took. I learned to accept every fall as an opportunity to study and not as a large defeat from which it was not possible to rise again. With that, I understood that there is an effect on the big picture in every component of my life, and in every component of my diet – from the herb to the main ingredient.

There is no such thing as "failure", only "what works" and "what doesn't work", and there is no end to the opportunities for learning. Falling has a value if you can learn from it. We cannot criticize ourselves when we make mistakes because they are the only things that are well and truly mine. If I give myself a chance, the mistake is not only an important lesson, but an important possibility that I had not seen before.

So when do we begin?

Now, today, this moment. The fact that you are interested in something new means you've already begun something. Everything that is different from what you know can bring change. They say that if you do today exactly what you did yesterday you can assume that nothing will change. I say that if you pay attention to something, and you change it, it may affect your health – and even if it's in the smallest way, then the change has already begun. It's true that paying attention by itself is not enough, but to widen it – that's a beginning. To pay attention to what's good for you and to what's not good for you is a stage that you cannot skip. Because it's not possible to isolate areas in your life definitively.

But first of all you need a plan. A plan that emanates from self-knowledge and from the understanding of the things that create motivation in us and the things that hold us back. We need to know what can hold us back as a lesson, and to prepare ourselves in advance. Part of the lesson is to understand that the struggle is what holds us back – whether it is paradigms or limiting beliefs. Sometimes it's like a tango: two steps forward – one step back. Sometimes we take a few steps forward at once, but at every step there is an option – forward or backward, the option of learning, or the option of changing, the option of feeling good, or the option of listening to what the body says when it doesn't feel good. The connection with and listening to the language of the body and the language of your world is the most important process. The results of this process are marginal benefits. The ability to be present and alert in the present is the main benefit.

It's very important to take breaks, to breathe and to experience the present. If your plan is attainable and you have set a goal and targets for yourself that are realistic within a realistic timeframe and are not stressful, take the time to celebrate every occasion that you overcome a small obstacle, an obstacle that is not necessarily something you can measure by your weight or the amount of bowel movements you have in a day. Sometimes you can celebrate a success over something or someone that was difficult to deal within the past, and that you have found a new way to do things that works for you – everything, in fact, that signals another milestone on the road to a healthy life.

To conclude, I hope that you have found food for thought and some inspiration. There is no single magic formula that is right for everyone. Each one of you has your own path to health. This path is full of ups and downs. With time the downs become ascents and they hurt less, and we learn to enjoy from the ascents and to gain from them. It is most important that you allow yourselves to be helped by those who are dear to you and your colleagues, and to hear the small signals and to listen to the signs as an opportunity for growing and flowering.

Conclusion

The chapters of this guide contain a great number of subjects connected in different ways to bowel diseases, and in particular to Colitis and Crohn's disease. It does not purport to be a single source of information for patients. The information about the disease changes and is updated all the time. I am full of hope that what appears in these pages will serve you during the course of your lives as patients, or as people living with patients, and will be a strong basis for every new piece of information. I recommend that you continue getting updates all the time, using books and the internet, researching and asking about any subject on which you want to focus. I believe that the book can provide some tools that will help you deal better with your disease, tools that will pass the test of time and its consequences.

Most importantly you should remember that you should never remain passive or ignore the disease. There is always something that can be done. You need to acknowledge your disease and learn to deal with it in your own way. As you've seen, there are a good number of ways and means to deal with the disease. The ball is definitely in your court. At the same time remember, at the end of the day every decision on the subject of your health is yours, not the doctor's or the therapist's. Consult everyone, but take the decision on your own.

Today I live in peace with Crohn's. I would call it a cold peace, or a ceasefire. I know my limits. I'm not really satisfied with them, but I acknowledge them. I make sure that I sleep eight hours a night, every night. My food comprises mainly eggs, fish, tahini, and various foods within the framework of the SCD. During calm times I eat more and try new foods, within reason, of course. I don't remember when I last ate out, although I don't give up on going out (yes, you can drink an infusion instead of coffee). I drink at least a liter of water a day, and do my best to play sport as much as my body will allow. I work full-time in a calm workplace, within my capacities. I take gentle iron pills and a multivitamin supplement. Once a month I do a comprehensive blood test in order to monitor my condition. If it's necessary I get a dose of iron or B12 either by infusion or injection. I'm visited from time to time by attacks of pain and diarrhea, and in response I acknowledge the fact that I'm having an attack, reduce my consumption of food, eat lots of soup and drink a lot of liquids, rest a lot, and from time to time use a little moxa. More than that, back massage and reflexology help me in calming the pain. Most importantly I remind myself that the attack is temporary and will pass. Once in a while I try a new treatment. Most recently it was yoga and guided imagery.

I have not stopped living my life. I surf, work, study and go out with my family and friends, and all within my capacity which changes at different times. I listen to my body and do not fight with it, and in this way I respond quicker to the disease. This is the reason that my recovery from attacks is quicker.

Remain optimistic, and keep your sense of humor. There many situations that Crohn's and Colitis patients go through, that it's possible and indeed desirable, to laugh at.

I wish you good health.

Tips for a good life

1. First of all, relax.
2. Invest time in learning what is good to eat and what is not.
3. Hot meals are good for the stomach, cold ones are not beneficial.
4. Quality is everything.
5. Where there is active inflammation, food = fuel for the inflammation.
6. Bodily fitness gives oxygen to the breath. Take advantage of the calm times in order to keep your fitness up.
7. You can always heal the body. True belief in that is the key to remission.
8. Learn to cook, or more correctly, learn to love cooking. In this way you'll learn to cook dishes that are tasty and good for your health.
9. Trust your sense of smell. Meat or fish that do not smell exactly like meat or fish will not strengthen your relationship with your digestive system.
10. Listen to your body before any other person – including your doctor.
11. Does it hurt a little? Rest and reduce your food – activity and food at a bad time will exact a price.
12. The sentence "There is nothing more important than health" takes on its meaning in the daily decisions of a Crohn's patient. You need to remember and to learn by heart that when we choose to eat something or do a particular activity, it can harm us.
13. Learn from your mistakes, this is the only way to get better.
14. A good state of mind is good for the health. Period.
15. Not every folk remedy is good.

16. When you ask people you will discover that when it comes to the stomach, everyone's a doctor.
17. What causes diarrhea in our healthy friends, will send you to hospital. Remember this on your next trip to the desert, South America, India or the gas station on the way to your vacation.
18. Routine is good, an irritated bowel doesn't like surprises.
19. Food is always preferable to food supplements, even in the form of juice.
20. Good sleep is essential for good health. Period.
21. Not every therapist who takes money knows what he is doing – you have been warned.
22. Step-by-step is the name of the game. Every change in your lifestyle or menu needs to be made slowly and with care, with great attention to the body's response. You can try new things, but gradually and carefully.
23. Laugh at the situations that Crohn's disease provides us with. There is a lot to laugh at.
24. Fall in love with your ability to surprise yourself – also in the bathroom.
25. An intestine that barks doesn't bite, but noise is a sign of things to come. Take this into account.
26. A healthy person will never feel his intestines, and therefore can never understand just what stomach pain is.
27. There is no such thing as too much drink (non-alcoholic) in a day.
28. Find a hobby – one that you will really love.
29. Spoil yourself with quality wipes.
30. It's not possible to overstate the importance of cleanliness and hygiene. You don't want to know what can develop in places where the sun doesn't shine.
31. Healthy and tasty food exists, it just demands more effort.
32. Make the most of the days and the good times to enjoy life.

33. Give your body the tools to deal with the inflammation.

34. Be true to yourself with regard to the habits that cause you to feel bad. Be stubborn in putting an end to them – bad habits die slowly, but they do die.

35. Remember – to balance the digestive system is like balancing a house of cards. The slightest breath of wind will force you to begin all over again.

36. Discover the rules of eating and lifestyle that help you to feel better, and keep them up. Every day that you feel good is another day that you distance yourself from the next attack.

37. Our emotional system does not end in the brain. Don't be afraid to investigate your spiritual side in order to solve health problems.

38. There is no point in fighting your body. You'll lose anyway.

39. If you don't listen to your body when it speaks quietly to you, you'll be in shock when it begins to shout.

40. When the bowel wants attention, give it to some.

41. Even the digestive system needs its rest.

42. Change big meals to continual small meals of quality food.

43. A dish that you have cooked or bought, and that you know after doing it that it won't be good for you – stop eating it. It doesn't matter what the level of investment was or the price of the portion. Health matters more than anything.

44. No matter what the state of your health, being busy always helps your internal feelings and your feeling of vitality, and this includes helping with chores around the house.

45. Do not discount any form of treatment, whether it's Chinese therapy, herbal therapy or a religious blessing. If you've decided to try it, it's important to invest in it, and to believe. Belief has power. No-one, including yourself can know what will contribute to your health until you try it. If you don't seek, you will not find.

46. It doesn't matter whether the disease started with a mental condition or not. Now that it exists, you need to treat it, and it's plain as daylight that your mental condition affects the condition of your health. Stress is bad!

47. Listen to the rhythm of the body, eat the right amount at the right time, go to sleep at a suitable hour, and do physical activities when the body can handle it.

48. Good intelligence decides wars. Therefore remember: monitoring, monitoring and monitoring. Keep to your blood tests and periodic tests at the doctor. The more information you gather the more you'll be able to take better decisions.

49. Health is more important than anything else. There is no task or place that you cannot leave, and it doesn't matter how much you are needed there.

50. Listen to everyone's advice but take the decision yourself.

Appendices

Appendix 1 – The anatomy of the digestive system

This appendix relates to the anatomical structure of the digestive system and is a summary of the description of the digestive system as it appears in The Ciba Collection of Medical Illustrations

A general explanation of the digestive system

The aim of the digestive system is to break down and absorb the food that we eat, and to produce energy through the elimination of waste from it. The system mainly comprises a hollow tube that begins at the pharynx and ends at the anus and includes a number of key organs, each with a different role in processing the food. The shape and action of this tube – the intestinal tract – varies according to position in the digestive system. Apart from the key organs, various glands are found in the system that help in breaking down the material, in its absorption in the circulatory system, and in their transfer to various tissues and their storage. The length of the human digestive system is about 7.5 meters and includes the main organs that are detailed in the paragraphs below.

Mouth

The mouth absorbs food. By chewing, the mouth completes the first breaking down of the food, mixes it with saliva and turns it into a pulp in preparation for swallowing. During the breaking down process a little of the components of the food is absorbed. The mouth includes the hard palate in the front part, and the soft palate in the back, teeth, tongue, muscles for chewing and salivary glands.

Esophagus

The esophageal canal begins at the pharynx (at the lower part of the throat), passes through the chest, via the diaphragm and connects to the stomach. It is about 25cm long and its role is to transfer the food from the pharynx to the stomach. The upper part of the esophagus is made of striated muscle and the lower part of smooth muscle. The connection between the lower esophageal muscles and the upper stomach muscles creates a kind of unidirectional sphincter that prevents any transfer from the stomach to the esophagus.

Stomach

The stomach is bean-shaped. The upper part it is connected to the esophagus and the lower part widens and connects to the duodenum (in the past this was known as the pyloric sphincter). The role of the stomach is to carry out the initial breaking down of the food by means of the stomach wall muscles which knead it, and the stomach acids which break it down chemically. The stomach walls are made up of fibers of smooth muscle. There is a network of longitudinal, horizontal and diagonal muscles that envelop the stomach, giving it strong walls that can withstand strong pressures.

Duodenum

The duodenum is horseshoe-shaped. The upper part is connected to the stomach. This passage between the duodenum and the stomach is the pyloric sphincter (see above). The lower part is connected to the large intestine. The role of the duodenum is to complete the process of breaking down the food that begins in the stomach. The walls of the duodenum are composed of two layers. The inner layer is composed of horizontal or circular smooth muscle fiber, and the outer layer is composed of horizontal fiber. Gall bladder secretions, or bile, and pancreatic secretions that are not essential for food digestion, drain at the duodenum.

The small intestine

The small intestine is a tube of about 5 meters long. Its main role is the absorption of food. The upper part is connected to the duodenum and its diameter is 3cm to 3.5cm. Its lower part is connected to the large intestine and its diameter is about 2.5cm. The small intestine has two layers: the inner layer is called mucosa (mucous) composed of circular smooth muscle. Above it is a layer of longitudinal muscle. Along the entire length of the small intestine, the inner mucosal layer is characterized by lots of circular folds whose purpose is to enlarge its surface absorption capacity. The wave-like contraction of the circular and longitudinal muscles in the small intestine moves the food forward (similarly to squeezing a tube of toothpaste). The food in the intestine moves at a speed of 1cm to 2cm a minute. These contractions are known as peristaltic movement. In a normal meal, the time it takes for the food to pass from the beginning of the small intestine to the large intestine varies between three to five hours. The small intestine secretes many enzymes that assist in the breaking down and absorption of food.

The end of the small intestine is known as the terminal ileum. It is typically a place where Crohn's disease appears. The connection between the small and large intestines is composed of spiral muscle called the ileocecal valve.

Colon

The colon is bow-shaped and its main role is to absorb water. The first part of the large intestine is connected to the small intestine and is called the ileal orifice [32]. Its terminal part ends at the rectum. Its length varies between 1.2m and 1.5 m. The large intestine is divided according to its position, into the ascending colon, the transverse

---

[32] Ileal orifice: www.medilexicon.com/medicaldictionary.php?t=63336

colon and the descending colon. The large intestine ends in the part called the sigmoid colon, which begins at the large intestine and descends to terminate at the rectum and the anus. The large intestine is made up of three of layers, the inner layer, known as mucosa, and two layers of smooth muscle.

Anus

The digestive system ends at the anus, a tube whose length is 3.5cm and through it, feces, the residue of the digested food, is expelled.

Appendix 2 – Blood tests [viii]

Test	Type	Values	Meaning	Description
ALK .PHOSPHAT [ATP]	Liver function	30 – 140	Malnutrition/liver disease/ anemia	Alkaline phosphate is an enzyme created in the liver and released into the blood. Low value: malnutrition and lack of protein. High value: various liver diseases.
ALT(GPT) [SGPT]	Liver function	5 – 45	Liver disease	Alanine transaminase is an enzyme created in the liver. High value: various liver diseases
AST(GOT) [SGOT]	Liver function	5 – 40	Infection/ anemia/ liver disease	Enzyme found mainly in heart muscle, and skeletal muscle and in the liver. High value: liver disease, anemia, infection. High values can occur after physical activity and pregnancy that do not necessarily indicate a problem.

Test	Type	Values	Meaning	Description
BILIRUB TOTAL [Bilirubin]	Liver function	0.3 – 1.2	Blood disease/ anemia/ bleeding/ liver disease	Bilirubin is the product of hemoglobin breakdown – a molecule that combines oxygen within red blood cells. High value: anemia, bleeding and liver disease.
IRON	Blood count	50 – 170	Malnutritio n/ anemia	Level of iron in the blood. Iron is essential for the creation of hemoglobin, the protein that carries oxygen in the blood, and the production of any other enzymes. Low value: usually a result of insufficient nutrition, a rise in consumption (as in pregnancy) or following bleeding.

Test	Type	Values	Meaning	Description
TRANSFERRIN	Blood count	200 – 380	Hematological problem	Protein that transfers iron from the blood to the bone-marrow, in order to create new blood cells
CRP [C-reactive Protein]	Chemistry	0 – 8	Active inflammation	Protein appearing in blood in high amounts when there is active inflammation.
ESR [Erythrocytes Sedimentation Rate]	Chemistry	2 – 20	Active inflammation	Blood sedimentation rate test. High sedimentation indicates inflammation.
WBC [White Blood Cells]	Blood count	4 – 10	Infection/ failure of the immune system	White blood cells are the main component of the immune system. Low value indicates a failure of the immune system, viral infection, or a response to immuno-suppressive drugs. High value indicates infection.

Test	Type	Values	Meaning	Description
NEUTROPHILS [Neut]	Differential	1.8 – 6.8	Infection/ blood production	White blood cells are responsible mainly for the destruction of bacteria. High value: bacterial infection. Low value : blood production problems, virus or response to chemotherapy
NEUTROPHILS % [Neut %]	Differential	46 – 68	Infection/ blood production	Neutrophil percentage of white blood cell count (WBC)
LYMPHOCYTES [Lymph]	Differential	4.5 – 6	Blood production / damage to the immune system/ infection/ cancer	White blood cells are responsible for the destruction of viruses and bacteria found in the body for an extended time. Low value: damage to the immune system. High value infection, cancer.

Test	Type	Values	Meaning	Description
LYMPHOCYTES % [Lymph %]	Differential	15 – 45	Blood production / damage to the immune system/ infection/ cancer	Lymphocyte percentage of white blood cell count (WBC)
MONOCYTES [Mono]	Differential	0.1 – 0.9	Blood production / damage to the immune system/ infection/ cancer	White blood cells are responsible for the destruction of bacteria, viruses and fungi. Low value: damage to the immune system, blood production problems, and can even indicate a cancerous process.
MONOCYTES % [Mono %]	Differential	2 – 9	Blood production / damage to the immune system/ infection/ cancer	Monocyte percentage of white blood cell count (WBC).

Test	Type	Values	Meaning	Description
EOSINOPHILS [Eos]	Differential	0 – 0.6	Allergy	White blood cells that fight infection and participate in the processes of allergy. High value: allergy, presence of parasites.
EOSINOPHILS % [Eos %]	Differential	0 – 6	Allergy	Eosinophil percentage of white blood cell count (WBC)
BASOPHILS [Baso]	Differential	0 – 0.2	Allergy	White blood cells that fight infection and participate in allergy processes. High value: allergy, presence of parasites.
BASOPHILS % [Baso %]	Differential	0 – 1.5	Allergy	Basophil percentage of the white blood cell count (WBC)

Test	Type	Values	Meaning	Description
RBC [Red Blood Cells]	Blood count	4.3 – 6	Blood production / anemia	White blood cells are responsible for combining oxygen from the lungs and go to body tissues. High value: blood production problems, an effect of smoking. Low value: anemia or heavy bleeding (normal values for women are slightly lower).
HEMOGLOBIN [Hb HGB]	Blood count	13.5 – 17.5	Anemia caused by lack of iron/ B12/bleeding/ chronic disease	Hemoglobin is a component of white blood cells, responsible for combining and release of oxygen and carbon dioxide. Low value: anemia(normal values for women are slightly lower).

Test	Type	Values	Meaning	Description
HEMATOCRIT [HCT]	Blood count	38 – 50	Anemia	Measure of the volume of red blood cells relative to the full blood count volume expressed as a percentage. Low value: anemia. High value: over-production of blood cells.

Test	Type	Values	Meaning	Description
MCV [Mean Corpuscular Volume]	Blood count	80 – 98	Anemia caused by lack of iron/ B12/ Folic acid	The average volume of a red blood cell. Low value: Anemia caused by lack of iron. High value anemia because of a lack of vitamin B12or folic acid.
MCH [Mean Cell Hemoglobin]	Blood count	25 – 35	Anemia	Average amount of hemoglobin in each single white blood cell. Low value: Anemia
MCHC [Mchc]	Blood count	32 – 35.5	Anemia	Concentration of hemoglobin. Low value: Anemia
PLATELETS [PLT]	Blood count	150 – 400	Bleeding/ blood-clotting problems/ bone-marrow problems	Platelets are responsible for one of the stages in blood-clotting. Low value: Blood-clotting disturbances and tendency to bleeding. High value: bleeding or bone-marrow disease.
MPV	Blood count	6.5 – 10	Platelet volume	Average volume of platelets. High value: Bone-marrow disease.

Test	Type	Values	Meaning	Description
RDW [Red Cell Distribution Width]	Blood count	11 – 14	Blood-production problems	A test that measures the differences between blood cells. Greater difference: Response to anemia. Over-production of red blood cells.
FERRITIN [Ferritin]	Blood count	21.8 – 275	Anemia caused by lack of iron	Ferritin is a combination of iron and protein comprising part of the body's iron reserves. Low value: Lack of iron.
FOLIC ACID	Blood count	3 – 34	Blood production / Anemia	Level of folic acid in the blood. Has a role in metabolism similar to vitamin B12. Lack of one of these can lead to a lack in the other. Low value. Abnormal production of red blood cells/ Anemia.

Test	Type	Values	Meaning	Description
VITAMIN B12	Blood count	157 – 1060	Anemia	Level of B12 in the blood. Essential for normal functioning of the nervous system and cells for utilization of folic acid. Low value: Anemia and degeneration of the nervous system.

Appendix 3 – Index of the seriousness of the disease

CDAI – Crohn's disease active index

CDAI is a research tool that reflects the activity of Crohn's disease over the past seven days.

You need to fill in the data for the past seven days and add them up.

You need to multiply the sum of each category by the multiplier that relates to it and add up all the results.

The meaning of the result:

- CDAI < 150 – A final result less than 150 reflects an inactive disease
- CDAI 150 – 450 – a final result of between 150 and 450 reflects a mild to moderate level of disease
- CDAI > 450 – A final result greater than 450 reflects a serious condition

Calculation form

X	Category	1	2	3	4	5	6	7	Total	Multiplier	Total X Multiplier
1	Number of soft or watery bowel movements per day									X 2	
2	Stomach pain index: 0: No pain; 3: Heavy pain									X 5	
3	General feeling 0: Good; 4: Very bad									X 2	
4	Complications: 1 point for every complication of the disease*									X 20	
5	Use of anti-diarrhea drug: 0: No; 1: Yes									X 30	
6	Value (complete) of deviation of Hct from the norm**									X 6	
7	Percentage of deviation of normal weight***									X 1	
										Total	

	Comments
*	Possible complications: temperature/ pain/ joint pain/ eye infection/ fissure/ fistula/ abscess/ skin problems
**	Hematocrit – Hct blood count, normal values: Men, 47%, Women, 42%. You can dispense with this value in the calculation
***	*100* x [(standard weight-actual body weight) / standard weight]. You can dispense with this value in the calculation

Site for automatic calculation of the results:

http://www.ibdjohn.com/cdai/cdaiOut.php

Additional details

http://en.wikipedia.org/wiki/Crohn's_Disease_Activity_Index

Appendix 4 – Links to websites

igutfeelings.com
twitter.com/iGutFeelings

Information on Crohn's disease

en.wikipedia.org/wiki/Crohns_disease
digestive.niddk.nih.gov/ddiseases/pubs/crohns/index.htm
www.nlm.nih.gov/medlineplus/crohnsdisease.html
www.webmd.com/ibd-crohns-disease/crohns-disease/tc/crohns-disease-topic-overview
www.crohns-disease-and-stress.com/index.html

Information on Colitis

en.wikipedia.org/wiki/Colitis
digestive.niddk.nih.gov/ddiseases/pubs/colitis
www.webmd.com/ibd-crohns-disease/colitis-guide/ulcerative-colitis-overview-facts

The Crohn's and Colitis Association of America

www.ccfa.org

Site for sharing information regarding Crohn's disease

www.crohnsonline.com

The story of coping with Crohn's disease

www.lessdoing.com/2013/05/06/how-i-overcame-crohns-disease/

Sources

Crohn's disease – General Information, Analysis and Tests:

- Davis – Christopher. Textbook of surgery. The biological basis of modern surgical practice. 1972 10th edition. 889-901.
- Marcus A. Krupp, Milton J. Chatton. Current diagnosis treatment. 1973. 328-9.
- C. Henry Kempe, Henry K Silver, Donough O'brien. Current pediatric diagnosis treatment. 1974. 432-3.
- R. A. Willis. The principles of pathology. 1950. 292.
- Harrison textbook of medicine. 1998, 14th edition.
- Frank H. Netter. The Ciba collection of medical illustrations, Volume 3 – A Compilation of Paintings on the Normal and Pathologic Anatomy of the Digestive System. 1975.106-110

Sources

[i] The Prince by Niccolo Machiavelli and W.K. Marriott (Kindle Edition – Feb 10, 2008)

[ii] The Power of Your Conscious Mind – Dr Joseph Murphy

[iii] The Power of Now – Eckhart Tall (Prague)

[iv] Manual of Freediving – Umberto Peltizzari, Stefano Tovagliert, Idelson Gnocchi

[v] Ideas and Opinions – Albert Einstein, Magnes Press – The Hebrew University

[vi] The Art of War – Sun Tsu

[vii] Dr Arieh Avini - Fools of Milk, On the damage caused by milk to health (2006) 114-128

[viii] Anaemia and Blood Tests:

- Marcus A. Krupp, Milton J. Chatton. Current diagnosis treatment. 1973. 256-9.

- Hematology. American Society of Hematology, Education Program Book. 2008. John W. Adamson. The Anemia of Inflammation/Malignancy: Mechanisms and Management. 159-165.

www.ingramcontent.com/pod-product-compliance
Lightning Source LLC
Chambersburg PA
CBHW071337280526
45787CB00001B/130